My Weigh

My Weigh

—⚲—

*What You Should Know About Weight Loss and
Maintenance Based on Medical Science*

Written and Illustrated by
Cully Narrie, MD

ISBN: 1517143551
ISBN 13: 9781517143558

This book is dedicated to my two daughters,
Elissa and Morgan,
who are the sweetest things in my life.

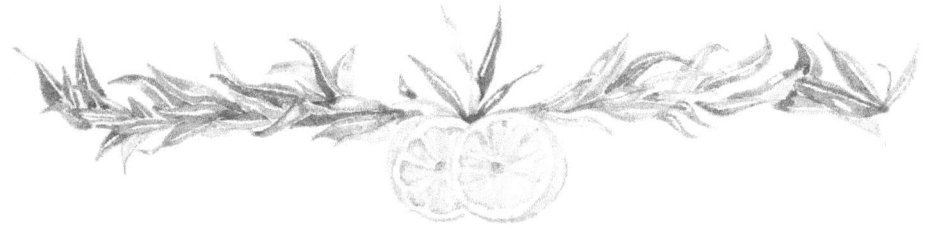

Contents

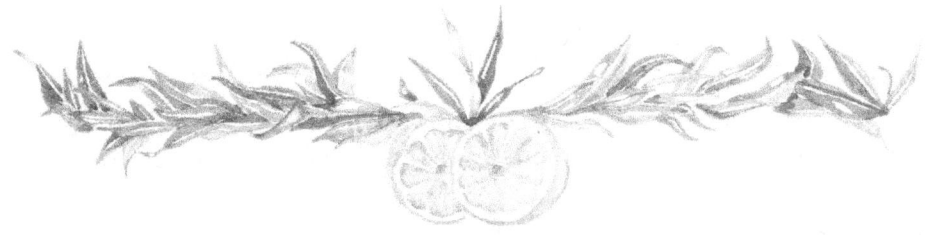

Introduction

I am a foodie. To say that I love food is an understatement. I am passionate about anything that has to do with food. Eating is only one element of the food pleasures that I enjoy. I often happily center my free time around cooking while watching the cooking channels. Shopping for food is one of the highlights of my day, and I do it every day. My library consists of over a hundred books on growing and preparing food. I attend the local farmers' market every Saturday to sample and marvel at the abundance of delectable fresh fruits, herbs, and vegetables. I love to meet ducklings, not because they are cute but because I can imagine the deliciousness of a potential Duck à l'Orange. I even gave birth to a chef (much to my delight).

My career as a doctor reflects my preoccupation with food. It has evolved to focus on the treatment of weight-related diseases and weight management. In 2014, I became board certified in obesity medicine. Attending conferences on obesity medicine is like going to rock concerts for me. To have a means of incorporating my obsession with food into my internal medicine practice is nothing short of a dream come true.

Obesity medicine is the study of the science; treatment; financial costs; and genetic, environmental, behavioral, and cultural factors of weight. "Obesity" is a medical term that is defined as a person having a body mass index of 30 or more. We doctors love numbers to define diseases. For example, if your blood pressure is 138/88, you don't have hypertension. But if it's 140/90, then…ahhh! You have hypertension! Or if your hemoglobin A1c is 6.4, you don't have diabetes. But if it's 6.5, then you are slapped with the label, medications, diet, and lifestyle of being a diabetic.

Body mass index is a similar numerical medical device, with strong medical and emotional implications. It is a calculation that reflects weight in relation to height. The formula is: (weight in pounds x 703/height in inches ^{2}). I have included a body mass index (BMI) chart in the appendix so you don't have to do the calculation in your head. If you are at or over the 30 mark, you are considered "obese." Nobody wants that label! If your body mass index is between 26 and 30, you are considered "overweight," another unsavory designation. The science of weight management is less restrictive for people age sixty-five and older. This group is not considered to be overweight until one's body mass index is over 30. In fact, some sources recommend that a BMI between 23 and 30 is healthy for this age group.

I dislike the term "obesity." Of all the medical labels for illnesses, this one to me is the most distasteful. Socially, it almost evokes a sense of crime. The understanding that many of my patients cannot control their weight without expert advice, as one with any medical illness would need, fuels my sense of dislike for this term. In medical circles, "obesity" is frequently used to describe the science of weight management. There is a board dedicated to prevention, treatment, and research for weight illness. It is called the Obesity Society (http://www.obesity.org). The term "obesity" is meant to be scientific and not degrading. It does not reflect lifestyle but rather a disease. And as with other diseases, the person who has obesity has to own it.

Diabetes, cardiovascular disease, and cancer require a person to take ownership if he or she is to survive. Obesity is not different. When compared to normal weight, obesity is associated with significantly higher death rates. Nearly one in five deaths in the United States is associated with this disease. Obesity leads to heart attack and stroke, diabetes, musculoskeletal disease, hormonal imbalance, neurologic disorders, and cancer, including cancer of the endometrium, breast, and colon. It is the visible killer. The bad news is that if you are overweight, you are on the path to these diseases. Ownership of your extra pounds is required to cure this disease. The good news is that obesity is curable with treatment and there are available resources to help.

So how can someone design a lifestyle that will allow that person to take ownership of his or her weight, achieve a healthy body, and be a happy foodie? It has to do with recognizing that we are all different in our dietary needs. One size does not fit all when it comes to weight management. Metabolism varies from individual to individual, as genetics design a unique pattern of metabolism for each person. Tastes differ, and health issues create needs for one person that may not be necessary for another. One may be taking essential medications that have a side effect of weight gain. A person may not be able to exercise because of arthritis. Age and gender affect our weight, as do cultural differences.

Achieving a healthy weight also requires developing realistic expectations, understanding the science behind weight management, and putting it into practice. I use this knowledge to treat my patients and to keep my own weight in check. When distilled, this science is easy to understand. But let's face it; it's a challenge to incorporate into everyday life. One must own the disease and take charge. My goal in this book is to provide the medical information you need to approach weight management to suit your individual needs. Whether you have a healthy weight and want to maintain it or whether you suffer from being overweight or have obesity, this book will help you to understand the science behind weight control. Basic and simple principles can be incorporated into your life and provide you with a framework for creating a lifestyle and a diet you will enjoy, which in turn will provide a basis for a lifelong healthy weight. This book has the information to guide you as you take ownership of every extra pound that you want to lose. And I will enjoy writing every sentence because, of course, it deals with food!

I

Metabolism

As a society, we have many barriers to successful weight management. There are busy schedules, economic restraints, tempting fast foods, and televisions and computers to lure us into inactivity (not to mention the cooking channels). We have been taught to use comfort foods to help relieve stress in our lives. There are medications that we need to take, but many are weight unfriendly. Furthermore, we are metabolically wired like cavemen and cavewomen. Don't think that you're going to sneak a cookie past your pancreas and have it go unnoticed! Your Paleolithic pancreas will shoot out insulin, a hormone that metabolizes the sugar in your blood, and turn that treat into fat storage for the cold winter of hibernation ahead before you even have a chance to reconsider the cookie. And as it drops, the rapidly falling blood sugar created by the surge of insulin will make you hungry for another cookie.

The pancreas is not the only organ in on the plan to hoard fat. The gut is another eager participant. There are hormones that are produced in the stomach and intestine to stimulate appetite. Ghrelin is one of these hormones. These hormones increase after diet-induced weight loss and cause increased hunger. It is not your imagination that you are hungrier when you're on a diet. Thanks to your hormones, you really are!

There are also hormones that suppress appetite. As you may have guessed, they decrease after you have lost weight, so you are hungrier. Since the brain has receptors for these hormones, it also works to maintain fat tissue as it is triggered to stimulate appetite by the gut hormones when you have lost weight through dieting. One study demonstrated that even after a year, a person will experience the tenacious behavior of these hormone adaptations that are left over from caveman physiology. It is unknown if the effects of these appetite-inducing hormones will eventually stabilize (Sumithran et al. 2011, 1597-1604). This may be one reason why it is difficult to maintain weight loss.

Is it any wonder that my patients come to me in a state of frustration because they can't lose extra pounds? I can't tell you how many times I've heard, "I'm exercising, watching my diet, and I still can't lose weight. Will you check my thyroid?" And how many times I've said, "It's not your thyroid."

The problem is that if you lose 5 pounds, your body will want it back. Thermogenesis, or the rate at which we burn calories, will change. It will become lower so your body can regain the lost 5 pounds. This process is called adaptive thermogenesis. Your resting metabolism will decrease by 15 calories a day for each 2.2 pounds that you lose. This adds up! The complex system of hormones and neurochemicals in the brain, gut, and glands is programmed to make this happen.

Even the protein hormone leptin, which appears to have a positive effect on weight loss through a reduction in hunger, can turn into a traitor. Leptin is produced by fat cells and acts on the brain to suppress appetite and increase energy output. One would think that the high leptin levels in people with high body fat would suppress the appetite and increase energy expenditure enough to keep the body at a healthy weight. Once again our ancestry recalls its sophisticated famine survival plan and turns on a switch that makes it insensitive to the appetite suppressant and energy-burning effects of leptin (Bray et al. 2008, 459–460).

In summary, a body that has a surplus of adipose tissue wants to keep that surplus of adipose tissue. A body that is lean will be sensitive to leptin and its appetite suppression and energy induction. The metabolic design is one that calibrates baseline energy needs to a lower setting in order to maintain a surplus of energy and it does so in the form of fat. The more you seesaw with your weight, the more you will regain pounds in adipose tissue. In the evolutionary scheme, our metabolism has not caught up with the energy needs of our culture. However, even though we may be overweight, we have the knowledge and technology to assist us with the means to construct changes in our diets and lifestyle to offset our metabolic woes.

Conor Weezil was one of my patients. He was a graduate student earning a degree in negotiations. At thirty years old, he was unhappy with his appearance. Being a very handsome man, he wanted to be even better looking. Conor was convinced that part of his ability to win over an audience in a negotiation would depend upon his appearance.

When he came to see me, he weighed 280 pounds, was 5 feet 9 inches tall, and his body mass index was 34. His blood sugars were mildly elevated and his blood pressure was high. Conor was also having a problem with fatigue due to sleep apnea. He had tried many diets and had spent a small fortune on meal substitutes. He needed me because he couldn't lose weight and keep it off. His diet history was a cycle of following a structured diet program, losing weight, then regaining his weight after about six months.

"Doc, I think there's something wrong with my metabolism," he said. "I do everything right. I follow my diet. I exercise. Then I stop losing weight. I get frustrated and go off the diet and gain my weight back. Maybe it's my thyroid."

"It's not your thyroid," I said. "But you are right. It is your metabolism. Have you ever tried to stick to a diet program for at least a year after you've achieved your goal weight?"

"I'm on a diet right now," he said.

"How long have you been on it?"

"Six months. I've lost 50 pounds, but it's no longer working," he replied.

"Conor, you won't like this," I said. "We can't negotiate with your metabolism. If you lose weight, your body will want it back. It's nature's way of protecting us from starvation. Your resting metabolism slows when you lose weight on a diet (Schwartz et al. 2010, 531–547). No wonder why you're at a standstill."

"How about a diet pill?" he asked.

"You need to stick to your diet and exercise program. Your weight has a metabolic set point. This is similar to a boiling point except instead of water turning into vapor, your calories turn into fat. It happens when the body reaches a BMI of about 30. Then it becomes very hard for one to lose weight. This is an evolutionary survival mechanism of prehistoric mankind that resulted from periods of famine and cold. In order to lose weight and keep it off, you need to fool your body into thinking you are in the hunter and gather mode. That is why frequent small meals and exercise are so important!"

"If you prescribe me the diet pill, I promise to make you look like a success, Doc. I will tell everybody what a wonderful doctor you are."

"I told you, Conor, you cannot negotiate with metabolism and you cannot negotiate with me. It's time you stick to healthy eating habits and exercise. Come back and see me when you've reached your goal weight. If you continue to seesaw with your weight, it's going to be harder for you to maintain your goal weight. Stay with your diet and don't go off it, even if you reach a plateau."

Six months later, Conor Weezil came back and was looking handsomer than ever. His blood sugars were normal, he was no longer suffering from high blood pressure, and his sleep apnea had resolved. He commented that persistence had been the key to his weight-management success and his good looks. Now he had to maintain his goal weight for at least a full year.

II

Calories

Kara Mel came to me because she needed to lose weight quickly and didn't know how. At twenty-eight years old, Kara was sitting in the enviable position of being one of the most popular newscasters on local TV. She was the weatherperson and had an uncanny ability to predict the weather accurately. Schools and businesses depended upon her. Parents would set their alarm clocks by her forecast because if Kara said snow was coming, they knew they would see snow, schools would be closed, and everybody could sleep in.

Over the past few years, Kara had slowly gained weight. Her weight gain became a problem when her silhouette began to block out the weather map and her audience could no longer see the areas that would be affected by a particular weather system. When the producer of the show threatened to fire her, Kara decided to come see me. At 5 feet 6 inches, she weighed 204 pounds. She had a body mass index of 32. We determined that Kara needed to lose a total of 44 pounds to achieve a body mass index of 25.

Since Kara wanted to lose weight quickly, I put her on a very-low-calorie diet of only 800 calories/day. I used a prepackaged meal plan that could only be obtained through a physician. This diet program needed to be medically supervised with weekly office visits because of the potential for metabolic and EKG abnormalities. According to my predictions, she would lose 4 to 8 pounds/week on this diet. After twelve weeks on the very-low-calorie diet, her calorie allowance would be slowly increased.

At three months, Kara had achieved her weight loss goal. The problem now would be keeping it off, because rapid weight loss can be associated with regaining of weight. Only 4 percent of dieters who follow a low-calorie diet maintain a weight loss over three to five years. In order to prevent this, Kara underwent extensive nutritional and physical activity training as well as habit restructuring.

When she returned for her one-year follow-up, she had good news. "I've kept my weight off and landed a spot on national television!" she told me. "I have to run because I'm meeting with my contract negotiator, Mr. Conor Weezil, this afternoon. Wish me luck!"

If you enjoy imagining your weight at 30 percent less than what it currently is, then you're in good company. Most people who want to lose weight set a goal for about 30 percent. It's great to aim for this amount. However, if you lose weight in smaller increments, your chances of lifelong success will be higher. Unless you are like Kara and need to lose weight quickly, try to shed 5 percent of your initial weight over the first three months. For example, if you weigh 300 pounds, shoot for a goal of 15 pounds over three months. A weight loss of just 5 percent reduces the risk of high cholesterol, hypertension, and diabetes!

Once you set your weight-loss goal, you need to figure out how many calories per day you need. Herein lies one of the fundamental principles of weight management: calories in = calories out. It's tricky because a variety of factors play into caloric need.

Men have more lean body mass than women and therefore have a higher energy expenditure and need to consume more calories than women of the same height (Tooze et al. 2007, 382).

Metabolic rate declines with age by approximately 2 percent per decade, or about 100 calories/day per decade after age twenty. So a person who is forty years old needs 200 less calories/day than a person who is twenty years old. Genetics also play a role in how many calories/day your body will need. People who fidget have a higher calorie need than those who are sedentary and don't squirm (Roberts et al. 2006, 651; Heymsfield et al. 2007, 346). All of these variables in metabolism result in an overall +/-20 percent difference in energy needs.

To get a basic idea of how many calories/day you need, multiply 12 by your weight in pounds. The average person needs about 12 calories/pound/day for weight maintenance. For example, if you weigh 200 pounds, your daily calories intake to maintain this weight would be 12 x 200 = 2,400 calories. If you consider the 20 percent variable, your calorie needs could be as high as 2,880 or as low as 1,920 calories/day.

So, if you're a twenty-year-old, two hundred pound male fidgeter with a family of skinny people, you can eat the 2,880 calories a day. If you're a fifty-year-old, two hundred pound sedate woman of the same height as the fidgety man, and you have people of weight in your family, you should take in no more than the 1,920 calories a day.

An easy way to figure out your daily needed caloric intake or total daily energy expenditure is to go to one of the websites that offers this calculation. Most of these take your gender and age into account. One such website is: nutritiondata.self.com/tools.calories-burned. MyFitnessPal.com is a popular website that helps you keep track of how many calories you need and take in during a day. ChooseMyPlate.gov has helpful information about calorie management.

If you want to lose 1 to 2 pounds a week, you should plan a deficit of roughly 500 calories/day or more if you have a sedentary lifestyle.

Being aware of calories is a basic ingredient in weight management. However, on an equal level is designing your diet around good calories. These will help reset your metabolic rate or BMI set point to maintain ideal weight. Many of my patients ask why simple carbohydrates (breads, pastas, rice, potatoes, sugary drinks, and sweets) are considered fat producing calories. Logically, one would think they are great short term energy boosters. The simple carbohydrates are excellent if you are immediately going to engage in an activity that will utilize calories, such as an exercise routine. However, if they can't find an energy burning outlet, they will drive themselves to the next level, which is being saved in the form of adipose (fat) tissue. Worse yet, the situation is compounded by the fact that simple carbohydrates make you hungry. Insulin (the hormone in our blood that turns the macronutrients to energy or fat), will fall quickly in response to simple carbohydrates. The quick fall makes you feel hungry. That's when the real trouble starts: you reach for the second cookie! Complex carbohydrates (legumes, foods high in fiber, and most vegetables, the exception of the starches), healthy fats (such as omega-3 and olive oil), and proteins take longer to metabolize, so insulin rises and falls at a slower rate than it does when responding to simple carbohydrates. Hunger signals are not sent off in response to this, so you eat less! That's why it's easier to lose weight when you avoid the simple carbs and go for the green, protein, or healthy fat instead.

III

Exercise!

Ellie P. Tickle was a single mom with two teenage children and a full-time job in the bakery at a local grocery store. Although she looked much younger than her age, she was fifty years old. With her metabolism slowing down and a few new items in the bakery, she had gained 30 pounds in the past year. Ellie was used to being able to eat anything she wanted and was stunned to find that cookies now made a difference.

Determined to get her youthful figure back to match her youthful face, she went on the South Beach Diet and lost 10 pounds but gained it back because she could not adhere to the tight restrictions of this program. Then she tried Weight Watchers and lost 20 pounds, but she found it tiring to constantly be counting points, so she gained the 20 pounds back. Finally, she decided to try the Volumetrics diet, which allows one to fill up with low-density foods, such as fibrous vegetables. Ellie liked this diet because it was not totally restrictive and she could have an occasional bakery item. However, when she lost 10 pounds and then continued to gain the weight back, she came to me for help.

"Are you exercising?" I asked.

"I hate exercise," she said. "Besides, I'm too tired and don't have time. I work full time and have two teenagers who need to be driven to basketball practices."

"You only have to exercise in ten-minute intervals to reap the benefits of exercise. Try walking at a brisk pace for ten minutes three times a day."

"I guess I could squeeze that in if you really think it will help. I have a treadmill in the basement or I could walk outdoors at lunch. I ought to do it," she said.

"I think the elliptical has your name on it," I told her.

One month later, Ellie came back and was impressed by how much more energy she had. "I'm dating a man who's younger than me by fifteen years," she said. "He works in the fish department. I feel that I can finally almost keep up with him. I'm going to increase my exercise."

At her six-month follow-up, Ellie was thrilled with her ability to keep weight off and her increased sense of well being. She was exercising by alternating the elliptical, treadmill, and cycle for a total of 150 minutes a week. Lifting weights was helping her maintain muscle mass as she lost pounds through calorie restriction.

I've heard it before: "I hate to exercise!"

Exercise helps our bodies in numerous ways. It lowers the risk of heart disease and stroke by lowering blood pressure and cholesterol (Kodama et al. 2009, 2024). Exercise lowers the risk of diabetes (Strasser et al. 2010, 397). It even lowers the risk of colon cancer, breast cancer, lung cancer, prostate cancer, pancreatic cancers, and endometrial cancer (Kushi et al. 2012, 30; Michaud et al. 2001, 921). Exercise helps to prevent osteoporosis and hip fractures. Physical activity improves energy levels and endurance, regular bowel function, fertility, immune system function, and joint motility (Strasser et al. 2010, 397). It also improves cognition and delays the onset of Parkinson's and Alzheimer's diseases. A recent report boasted about the positive therapeutic effect that exercise has on stable ischemic heart disease and advised that it should be prescribed routinely (Boden et al. 2014, 905–911). Exercise results in reduced abdominal girth, improves sleep, and helps with weight loss and weight maintenance (Rowe et al. 2014, 798–810). Physical activity spares loss of muscle during weight loss.

It also improves mood and facilitates adherence to a healthy eating program.

There are three types of exercise that you engage in every day, whether you hate them or not. The first is resting energy expenditure. This burns approximately 60 percent of our daily calories. The second is the thermic effect of meals. This accounts for approximately 10 percent of our daily calories and is the energy needed for digestion. Protein and alcohol fare the best for diet-induced thermogenesis, giving protein the highest score for the macronutrients. Carbohydrates and fats utilize less percentage of energy for digestion, which also contributes to a diminished feeling of fullness.

The third is energy expenditure from physical activity, which includes structured exercise as well as another physical activity called NEAT, or nonexercise thermogenesis. About 30 percent of our calories are spent on physical-activity energy each day. NEAT is a type of energy expenditure that takes into account weight, gender, body composition, and daily nonstructured exercise activities such as standing upright, sitting, fidgeting, and walking. It also includes the energy you expend at your occupation. NEAT energy expenditure can result in up to 2,000 calories/day beyond the basal metabolic rate (Villablanca et al. 2015, 509–519). Energy from physical activity, whether it is through structured exercise or NEAT, is important. It varies from person to person and can determine in part why two people who take in the same amount of calories may have different weight gain.

Total daily physical energy expenditure can be measured by using the double-labeled water technique, or one can use a triaxial accelerometer. However, I don't recall ever seeing one of these devices displayed for public use. Pedometers are handy little gadgets that will provide a measurement of physical activity. Many companies have designed measuring devices to keep track of your exercise accomplishments, calories, and even how you sleep. If technology fits into your life, you may enjoy using them. By knowing how many calories are burned in a particular activity, you can estimate your caloric expenditure through physical activity. Below is a list of common exercises and the calories burned (for a 154 pound 5 foot 10 inch man):

- **HIKING**: 370 calories/hour
- **LIGHT GARDENING/YARD WORK**: 330 calories/hour
- **DANCING**: 330 calories/hour
- **GOLF** (walking and carrying clubs): 330 calories/hour
- **BICYCLING** less than 10 miles/hour: 290 calories/hour
- **WALKING** at 3.5 miles/hour: 280 calories/hour
- **WEIGHT TRAINING** (general light workout): 220 calories/hour
- **STRETCHING**: 180 calories/hour
- **RUNNING OR JOGGING** at 5 miles/hour: 590 calories/hour
- **BICYCLING** more than 10 miles/hour: 590 calories/hour
- **SWIMMING FREESTYLE SLOW LAPS**: 510 calories/hour
- **AEROBICS**: 480 calories/hour
- **WALKING** at 4.5 miles/hour: 460 calories/hour
- **HEAVY YARD WORK** such as chopping wood: 440 calories/hour
- **WEIGHT LIFTING** with vigorous effort: 440 calories/hour
- **BASKETBALL** (vigorous): 440 calories/hour

Based upon large observational studies, medical evaluation prior to starting an exercise program is not necessary for asymptomatic people at low risk for coronary artery disease. However, if you have cardiovascular disease, you should have a preexercise evaluation. Cardiovascular disease risk includes hyperlipidemia, hypertension, smoking, diabetes, and history of premature myocardial infarction or sudden cardiac death in a first degree relative under age sixty. Having one or more of these conditions is an invitation to speak with your doctor before starting to exercise.

The standard exercise prescription is based upon frequency, intensity, time, and type of activity. Assuming your doctor has not put limitations on your ability to exercise, you should aim for a weekly goal of 150 minutes of moderate aerobic activity (such as walking) or 75 minutes of vigorous activity (such as jogging). Add in your resistance exercise two to three times a week. There is no data that demonstrates the superiority of one type of exercise over another, although a combination of resistance and aerobic is beneficial in increasing muscle mass, decreasing insulin resistance, and increasing cardiovascular fitness (Pate et al. 1995, 402).

Another type of exercise is high-intensity interval training, which involves intermittent brief sessions of high intensity workout. High-intensity interval training has been shown to improve cardiovascular fitness in the short term (Wisloff et al. 2009, 139). The long-term health benefits of high-intensity interval training are not known.

Exercise can be successful and has beneficial effects even if performed in short intervals during the day. As Ellie was told, even a ten-minute exercise session will make a difference.

Despite what you may have heard, achievement of heart rate goal is not necessary (Bosquet et al. 2008, 709). To maintain goal weight after weight loss, you may have to exercise sixty minutes each day because of the change in your metabolism (Wadden et al. 2011). Some studies show that one cannot lose weight with exercise alone. Exercise aids in weight maintenance by preserving and increasing muscle mass, which allow you to metabolize your calories more efficiently. It helps with regulating your metabolism so that once your goal weight is achieved, you can maintain it.

Year 1 of the Look AHEAD (Action for Health in Diabetes) study showed increased weight reduction in people who exercised (brisk walking or similar aerobic activity) 50 minutes/week and gradually progressed to 175 minutes/week over six months. Year 4 of the Look AHEAD study demonstrated that people who exercised were able to keep weight off (Wadden et al. 2011). The National Weight Control Registry is testimony to the results of this study. This is a registry of about 10,000 people who have managed to each lose 30 pounds and keep it off for 5.5 years. They exercise with approximately 60 to 90 minutes of moderate activity daily, burning about 400 calories/day. The most frequent activity is walking.

A study of 34,000 middle-aged women demonstrated that high levels of moderate to vigorous physical activity, approximately sixty minutes/day, were required to maintain normal body weight (Bassik and Manson 2005, 1193–1204). Another study that supports the need for exercise was recently published. Here it was reported that in the past two decades, men who reported no leisure-time physical activity increased from 19 percent to 52 percent. Women's lack of physical activity increased from 11 percent to 43.5 percent. To no surprise, both waist circumference and BMI increased significantly in both men and women. The surprise was that the magnitude of the increases was associated with the level of leisure-time physical activity but not with caloric intake (Ladabaum et al. 2014, 717–727).

Even in people with a normal BMI, waist circumference is an independent predictor of mortality and morbidity (Koster et al. 2008, 2105–2120). Having a prominent abdomen is like having a storage of toxic waste. If you have a lot around the middle, you need to lose it.

The liver is key to fat metabolism. When you have excess energy intake and the liver can no longer metabolize the fatty acids, you will get a fatty liver. Excess fat will also be deposited around the heart, blood vessels, and visceral region. When you gain weight in your middle, it is a reflection that these processes are occurring. As you can imagine, these deposits are not good for your health.

Normal weight women and overweight women and men have become more "abdominally obese." This trend is especially prominent in young women. The reason for this is a lack of physical activity. Adipose or fat tissue secretes potential inflammatory substances that may lead to the development of chronic diseases, especially respiratory diseases for reasons unknown.

Inside your gut are microbiota. These are organisms, bacteria for the most part, that play a role in energy harvest, storage, and expenditure. These gut flora have been shown to differ in obese and lean humans, and they change rapidly in response to dietary factors. Recent research has proposed that these tiny organisms residing in our intestines are critical for our uptake of nutrients, energy regulation, and weight and metabolic disorders.

When someone changes from a low-fat to a high-fat, high-sugar diet, the gut microbes undergo a rapid shift and this only takes one day! This dietary change has been shown to induce obesity if it occurs repeatedly. The gut microbes, when exposed to a large fries and a coke, will change and cause increased permeability of the intestinal wall. Resulting inflammation, insulin resistance, fat-cell hyperplasia (growth), and decreased function of the pancreas will cause a person over time to develop the metabolic syndrome, a condition characterized by three of the following: abdominal obesity, high blood sugar, hypertension, low HDL cholesterol and elevated triglycerides—not a pleasant scenario. You gut has evolved into a toxin tank.

Research is exploring ways to help reconstruct the tiny gut microbes into a healthy environment of weight-friendly bacteria. Diet will change the flora. Antibiotics are being explored as another way of manipulating the bacterial population, but no data is available at this time. Probiotics, such as the lactobacillus found in yogurt, are living microorganisms that offer therapeutic effect through replenishing a healthy environment (Di Baise et al. 2012, 22–27).

IV

Diets

In addition to disliking the word "obesity," I dislike the word "diet." It makes me uncomfortably hungry just to hear the word. As someone who loves food, I prefer to not use the term "diet" when referring to a structured eating plan. When I think about being on a "diet," feelings of misery and starvation are conjured up in this foodie's mind. A healthy eating plan should provide a structure in which one can enjoy food and at the same time feel better, improve health, improve self-esteem, and enhance life.

In this chapter, I will describe some of the most well known and studied diets that don't require starvation in order to be successful weight control measures. They include the Atkins, South Beach, Zone, Biggest Loser, Jenny Craig, Nutrisystem, Volumetrics, Weight Watchers, Ornish, and Mediterranean diets. You may decide you want to engage one of these or create your own unique eating plan.

In a medical study, eight diets were examined and compared. The conclusion was that the low-carbohydrate and low-fat diets fared slightly better than other diets, but essentially no one program was better than another regarding weight loss (Johnston et al. 2014, 923–933). The study compared the low-carbohydrate diets against the macronutrient (or balanced) diets and the low-fat diets. Adkins, South Beach, and Zone were the low-carbohydrate diets. The Biggest Loser, Jenny Craig, Nutrisystem, Volumetrics, and Weight Watchers were the macronutrient diets. The low-fat diets were the Ornish and Rosemary Conley. The difference in weight loss between the individual diets was minor and unimportant to those interested in losing weight!

A diet low in simple carbohydrates can be socially, culturally, and simply difficult to follow because we all like carbs and they are everywhere. Evidence currently supports advantages of this diet in terms of rapid weight loss and improvement in cardiovascular parameters. Simple carbohydrates have the problem of being rapidly metabolized and leaving us hungry sooner than would consumption of protein or foods with fat or complex carbohydrates. Since you don't get as much bang for your buck with simple carbohydrates, they should be limited or you will be inundated with excess calories from trying to stay satiated.

I recommend that you choose a personalized health focused diet that you like and think you can adhere to in order to reach your weight goals. You should decide what diet to follow based upon the foods you most enjoy. You may need to consider medical conditions that affect you. For example, if you are diabetic, you would benefit from a diet low in simple carbohydrates. If you have high cholesterol, you should follow a diet that's low fat and low in simple carbohydrates (Nordmann et al. 2013, 285–293). A study showed that a low carbohydrate diet of less than 4 grams/day of nonfiber carbohydrates (in other words, simple carbohydrates) resulted in greater improvements in body composition, HDL cholesterol levels, triglycerides, and estimated ten-year coronary risk (Bazzano et al. 2014, 309–318).

For those with concerns about heart health, another recent study showed that eating fish appears to be beneficial in preventing myocardial infarction. Having fish four times a week with each serving averaging around 100 grams or approximately 3.5 ounces offers protection. It is thought that this occurs because the omega-3 fatty acids in fish are readily absorbed into plasma lipids, resulting in a higher plasma concentration of omega-3 fatty acids. They therefore provide even more protection than omega-3 supplements, which aren't absorbed as well (Leung et al. 2014, 848–857).

Low-carbohydrate diets are gaining popularity because of the rapid weight-loss advantage and the additional benefit of decreased cardiovascular risk. If you decide to go on a low-carbohydrate diet, you need to understand the difference between simple and complex carbohydrates. One is bad for weight management and one is good, with simple being bad and complex being good. Simple carbohydrates are different than complex carbohydrates, as they are foods that are very easily digested, can lead to excessive weight gain, and immediately raise the blood sugar level. Complex carbohydrates are foods that take longer to digest and gradually raise the blood sugar level. The slower rise in blood sugar results in an efficient use of calories for energy requirements and helps maintain a sense of fullness. Additionally, complex carbohydrates contain fiber and vitamins, and should not be neglected in your diet.

Simple carbohydrates include bread and bread products such as waffles, bagels, muffins, tacos, and noodles. Other simple carbohydrates are starchy vegetables such as potatoes (including sweet potatoes), rice (including brown rice), and peas. Simple carbohydrates can also be found in some fruits. You should be careful to limit your intake of fruits, even though they contain vitamins and fiber, and can be healthy. Candy, cookies, cereal, popcorn, sugar, honey, syrup, and jam are also simple carbohydrates. Milk and dairy products contain simple carbohydrates and should be limited to skim milk or nonfat dairy.

Complex carbohydrates include green vegetables, high fiber grain, and legumes such as beans. Low-calorie complex carbohydrates, such as green leafy vegetables, are great and can be eaten as desired. Since grains and legumes have high caloric content, they should be limited.

Fats are part of a healthy diet. Olive oil is considered a good fat. It is a MUFA, or type of fat that is known as a mono-saturated fat. This type of fat is also found in avocados, nuts, and the omega-3 fish oil in salmon, and other fatty fish. It helps lower your cholesterol. Not only does it lower lipids, but it also is full of polyphenols, which are antioxidants that protect your cells from inflammation and damage. Consuming more than four tablespoons a day of olive oil can significantly lower your risk of having a heart attack or stroke. I don't recommend this much olive oil because at 119 calories/tablespoon, it is high in calories. However, consuming it at even lower doses offers benefits, especially if complemented with a daily serving of a fatty fish such as salmon, rainbow trout, pacific halibut, or tuna.

Balanced Diets

These diets focus on fulfilling the USDA requirements for a healthy diet, with 45 to 65 percent carbohydrates, 10 to 35 percent protein, and less than 35 percent fats (Medline Plus. Diets. 2015). Carbohydrates have 4 calories/gram, protein has 4 calories/gram, alcohol has 7 calories/gram, and fat has 9 calories/gram. Examples are the Volumetrics, Biggest Loser, Jenny Craig, Nutrisystem, Mediterranean, and Weight Watchers diets.

Volumetrics Diet

This diet consists of 55 percent carbohydrates, 10 to 35 percent protein, and 20 to 35 percent fats. It fills you up with foods that are low-density energy foods. These foods are low in calories but high in volume. For example, a pound of carrots, which are low density, contains as many calories as an ounce of peanuts, which are high density.

The diet divides foods into four categories: from lowest density to highest. You will eat mostly from the low-density categories. Three meals and two snacks are basic to the plan. The advantage of this diet is that you will not feel hungry and it's not expensive. It doesn't ban any particular food group, so you can adjust it to your liking, and because of this, it is a lifetime-friendly diet.

Biggest Loser Diet

This diet consists of 50 percent carbohydrates, 30 percent protein, and 20 percent fats. It emphasizes eating regular meals of fruits, vegetables, lean protein sources, and whole grains. The Biggest Loser program requires portion control, keeping a food journal, and exercising. The advantage of this diet is that it is not inconveniently restrictive on foods. You should not have a problem with consuming hunger pangs because there is a fiber- or protein-packed meal or snack every few hours. Exercise is central to this diet.

Jenny Craig

This diet consists of 50 to 60 percent carbohydrates, 10 to 35 percent protein, and less than 20 to 35 percent fats. The program includes prepackaged meals and recipes, and weight loss occurs through calorie restriction. When on the Jenny Craig Diet, you eat three meals and two snacks a day. The advantage of this program is that you get a weekly one-on-one session with a Jenny Craig consultant. Also, a special diabetes diet is available. However, you pay for it. The initial registration fee is about $400 and a week's worth of Jenny's Cuisine is $100. If you stay 5 pounds within your goal weight for a year, you will get half your registration fee back.

Nutrisystem

Nutrisystem is a diet that consists of prepackaged food with a few additional store-bought items such as fruits, vegetables, dairy, and proteins including chicken and fish. On this diet, you will eat five to six times a day and should not feel hungry. It is convenient because you don't have to count calories and it tells you when and what to eat. Over 150 foods are offered on this plan, which costs between $300 and $340 for twenty-eight days, not including store-bought items. Thirty minutes of daily exercise is encouraged for optimal weight loss.

Mediterranean Diet

The Mediterranean diet consists of 50 percent carbohydrates, 10 to 35 percent protein, and 20 to 35 percent fats. It includes a high level of monounsaturated fat relative to saturated; moderate consumption of red wine; moderate consumption of dairy products mostly in the form of cheese; high consumption of fruits, legumes, vegetables and grains; and a relatively low intake of meat.

This diet has been found to be associated with improved health through reductions in overall mortality, cancer mortality, the incidence of Parkinson's disease, cognitive decline, Alzheimer's disease, and cardiovascular mortality (Sofi et al. 2008, 1344). The diet requires calorie restriction for weight loss. If you enjoy cooking, this is a great diet for you, and you can indulge in a wine that will complement your food

Weight Watchers Diet

With this diet, no food is off limits. It focuses on lifestyle change and creating healthy eating habits. This diet uses a point-based system (PointsPlus) to create a framework for a calorie deficit of approximately 1,000 calories a day. There is an online program as well as an in-person program. Although it has a cost associated with it, Weight Watchers is paid for by some insurance companies.

Low-Carbohydrate Diets

Low-carbohydrate diets include either 60 to 130 grams of carbohydrates/day or 0 to less than 60 grams of carbohydrate/day if you want a very low-carbohydrate diet. These diets cause significant weight loss in the first two weeks that you are on the diet, where weight loss occurs from the breakdown of glycogen and fluid loss. These diets are more effective than low-fat diets in the short term but not in the long term at twelve months. Low-carbohydrate diets may be especially helpful in people with diabetes and/or high triglycerides (Freedman 2001, 1S-40S). A diet low in simple carbohydrates will help to raise you HDL, which is the protective cholesterol. It will also help to lower triglycerides. Examples of low-carbohydrate diets are the Zone, Atkins, Paleo, and South Beach diets.

Zone Diet

This diet consists of 40 percent carbohydrates, 30 percent protein, and 30 percent fats. If you like structure, you may enjoy this diet. It requires eating on strict schedule with breakfast within one hour of waking up and snacks and meals every five hours. One must also measure out foods. No food is completely off limits; however, foods high in simple carbohydrates, fats, and cholesterol are considered unfavorable.

Atkins Diet

This diet consists of 6 percent carbohydrates, 35 percent protein, and 59 percent fat. This is a high-fat diet with severe carbohydrate restriction. It advises avoidance of vegetables, fruits, cereals, breads, and most dairy products, except for two small green salads a day.

Paleo Diet

This diet consists of 23 percent carbohydrates, 38 percent protein, and 39 percent fats. It tries to imitate the way our ancestors ate when they were gathering and hunting. This diet goes back over ten thousand years and focuses on animal proteins and fats, eliminating dairy and grains. The disadvantage of this diet is that it is difficult to follow because it restricts food groups. An advantage is that you won't feel hungry because you eat plenty of protein and fiber.

South Beach Diet

The South Beach Diet consists of less than 45 to 65 percent carbohydrates, 10 to 35 percent protein, and 25 to 35 percent fats, with a decrease in fat percentage to less than 35 percent in the second phase. It unfolds in three phases, each one becoming less restrictive. This diet replaces bad carbohydrates, or the simple carbs, with good carbohydrates, or complex carbs. It also replaces bad fats with good fats. You eat three meals a day with two snacks and one high-protein dessert (such as mousse). The advantages are that there is no calorie counting or keeping track of fat grams or grams of carbohydrate. Satiety is also not a problem on this diet. The main disadvantage is that is requires willpower because it is restrictive.

Low-Fat Diets

A low-fat diet limits one to no more than 30 percent fat in your daily food intake. If food "melts in your mouth," it likely has fat in it. Eating no more than 30 percent of your calories in fat is the equivalent of about 33 grams of fat for each 1,000 calories. You can use the nutrition information on food packages to calculate this. The Ornish diet is a low-fat diet.

Ornish Diet

This is a very low-fat diet that helps you to lose weight and maintain heart health because you're eating fewer calories and consuming low levels of fat. This is a high-carbohydrate diet that is essentially vegetarian. Meats, eggs, oils, nuts, seeds, high-fat fruits and vegetables, and alcohol are forbidden. There are disadvantages of this diet, in that it restricts foods such as nuts and seeds that are important to heart health and that it is difficult to follow over the long term. Also, this diet results in hunger because of the extremely low-fat content.

High-Protein Diets

High-protein diets have the advantage of sparing muscle loss and increasing satiety. These programs utilize proteins of high biologic value. You get a lot of bang for your buck with protein, and protein helps to reduce your food intake through increased satiety related to diet-induced thermogenesis (Westerterp 2004, 1–5).

Protein Sparing Modified Fast

A diet called the Protein Sparing Modified Fast is helpful for diabetics with a BMI of 30 or higher. It is also an effective diet for diabetics with a comorbidity such as hypertension, sleep apnea, osteoarthritis, or fatty liver, who also have a BMI of 27 or higher. People who want to avoid diabetes and who also have either a BMI of 30 or more or a BMI of less than 27 with comorbidities (such as hypertension, sleep apnea, and hyperlipidemia) will benefit from the weight loss associated with this diet.

This program offers rapid weight loss over the first six months, leading to an average weight reduction of 46.2 to 84.9 pounds. Since it can cause electrolyte imbalance, dehydration, and liver and kidney damage, it must be supervised by a physician (Chang and Sangeta 2014, 557–565). High-protein diets may also lead to an increase in urinary calcium excretion because they cause an acid-producing load. Elevated urinary calcium can lead to kidney stones.

Very-Low-Calorie Diets

Another diet category is the very-low-calorie diet. This is the weight-loss program that I prescribed for Kara Mel because she needed to lose weight quickly or lose her job. Having extremely low-energy consumption, this plan offers 500 to 800 calories/day. It consists of prepackaged food that contain the recommended daily requirement of minerals, trace elements, fatty acids, vitamins, and proteins. In some very low-calorie diets, carbohydrates may be entirely eliminated. This diet can only be prescribed by a physician and must be medically supervised, with a checkup every two weeks. Resulting in about a five-pound weight loss/week and potential metabolic disturbances, it is only prescribed for twelve weeks. Side effects include fatigue, constipation, hair loss, thin skin, nausea, diarrhea, and gallstones.

You should only consider this program if your BMI is 30 or more or if your BMI is between 27 and 30 and you have a comorbid condition (diabetes, hypertension, hyperlipidemia, sleep apnea, or other serious medical illness caused by your weight). A disappointing aspect of this diet is that weight regain is common.

V

Medications and Herbal Supplements

Medications can facilitate your weight loss. Unfortunately, there are many more medicines that increase weight than there are those that enable weight loss. I have listed some of the weight-unfriendly medications below, indexed by disease.

Weight-Unfriendly Medications

Diabetes:

- Glucotrol (Glipizide), Diabeta (Glyburide), Amaryl (Glimperide)
- Prandin (Repaglinide), Starlix (Nateglinide)
- Actos (pioglitazone)
- Regular Insulin, Humalog Insulin (Insulin Lispro), Novolog (Insulin Aspart), Apidra (Insulin Glulisine), NPH, Levemir (Insulin Detemir), Lantus (Insulin Glargine)

Hypertension:

- Beta Blockers: Lopressor (Metoprolol), Tenormin (Atenolol), Trandate (Labetalol), Coreg (Carvedilol) (which is the least likely to cause weight gain out of this group)

Diuretics:

- Hydrochlorothiazide, Spironolactone (this group is more weight friendly than the beta blockers)

Antipsychotics:

- Thorazine (Clozapine), Zyprexa (Olanzapine), Risperdal (Risperidone), Geodon (Zirasidone), and Abilify (Aripiprazole) are the least weight gaining in the group

Antidepressants:

- Paxil (Paroxitine), Prozac (Fluoxetine), Elavil (Amitriptyline), Seroquel (Quetiapine)

Anticonvulsants:

- Depakote (Valproic Acid), Tegretol (Carbamazepine), Lithium

Others:

- Neurontin (Gabapentin)
- Antihistamines, including Benadryl (diphenhydramine)

Weight-Friendly Medications

Diabetes:

- Metformin (has additional advantages of decreasing visceral intra-abdominal fat, improving fatty liver, and counteracting the

weight gain that can occur with antipsychotic drugs, and if you have polycystic ovarian syndrome, it also helps this)
- Byetta (Exenatide), Victoza (Liraglutide)
- Symlin (Pramlinitide)
- Invokana (Canagliflozin)
- Januvia (Sitagliptin) and Onglyza (Saxagliptin) are weight neutral

Hypertension:

- ACE Inhibitors: Prinivil (Lisinopril), Capoten (Captopril)
- Angiotensin Receptor Blockers: Cozaar (Losartan), Diovan (Valsartan), Benicar (Olmsartan)

Antidepressants:

- Wellbutrin (Bupropion), Serzone (Nefazodone), and Zoloft (Sertraline) are weight neutral

Antipsychotics:

- Geodon (Ziprasidone) and Moban (Molindone) are weight neutral.

Drugs Designed to Assist in Weight Loss

Pharmacotherapy is limited to those with a BMI greater than 27 who have comorbidities (hypertension, hyperlipidemia, diabetes, sleep apnea, and osteoarthritis) or those with a BMI greater than 30 with or without obesity-related risk factors (National Institute of Health 2000). Drug therapy serves as an adjunct to exercise and calorie restriction, and should not be relied upon as a single therapy for weight loss.

Three drugs have recently been approved by the FDA for use in weight loss: Lorcaserin (Belviq), Naltrexone SR/Bupropion SR (Contrave), and Phentermine HCl/Topiramate (Qsymia). These three medications act in different ways.

Lorcaserin (Belviq) is a cousin of Prozac (Fluoxetine), Zoloft (Sertraline), and the group of SSRI drugs. In fact, you should be cautious taking Lorcaserin if you're taking an SSRI, Wellbutrin (Bupropion), or Effexor (Velantifine) and should speak with your doctor about possible interactions. Lorcaserin acts in the brain by causing an increased sense of satiety, thereby acting as an appetite suppressant. Side effects include headache, dizziness, nausea, and constipation. At one year, you can expect to lose 5 percent of your body weight or more (Bays 2009, 1429–1445).

Naltrexone SR/Bupropion SR (Contrave) acts on the reward center of the brain to reduce craving and habit power. It stimulates and inhibits various pathways of the central nervous system. Exactly how the combination causes weight loss is not completely understood. Contraindications include a history of seizures, psychiatric illness, or drug or alcohol misuse in the previous twelve months. Cardiovascular, cerebrovascular, hepatic, and kidney disease are also contraindications. Side effects include nausea and constipation. As are the other two weight-loss medications mentioned here, this drug is teratogenic and should not be taken during pregnancy. Change in body weight can be expected to be 5 percent or more after twelve months.

Phentermine HCl/Topiramate (Qsymia) acts as an appetite suppressant by stimulating the release of norepinephrine in the brain. The Topiramate (Topamax) in it changes taste perception. The Conquer study (The Lancet 2011, 1341-1352) demonstrated that this drug can improve waist circumference, reduce blood pressure, and lower triglycerides and cholesterol. Contraindications to this medication include glaucoma, hyperthyroidism, and pregnancy or nursing (it is teratogenic and can cause congenital malformations). The Lancet study showed that 37 percent of people taking 7.5 mg/46.0mg Qsymia lost 10 percent of their body weight in 56 weeks. The higher dose of Qsymia at 15.0mg/92.0mg offered even more benefit with 48 percent of the study participants losing 10 percent of their body weight in 56 weeks.

Liraglutide (Saxenda) was approved by the FDA in 2014 for the treatment of obesity. The dose is 3.0 mg daily instead of the 1.2 mg or 1.8 mg given in diabetes (in which the drug in known under the brand name Victoza). You should not use Liraglutide if you have a history of thyroid C-cell tumor. The most common side effects are low blood sugar, diarrhea, headache, fatigue, abdominal pain, and dizziness. The cost is about $400.00/month.

Another medication—and one that is not frequently used because its side effects include abdominal cramps, expelling gas, and oily discharge from the rectum—is Orlistat. Orlistat acts on gut signaling by inhibiting gastrointestinal absorption. It can be purchased over the counter without a prescription.

One of the problems with Belviq, Contrave, and Qsymia is that they are costly. A thirty-day supply of Belviq is about $107, a thirty-day supply of Contrave is about $70, and a thirty-day supply of Qsymia is $181. Phentermine, an appetite suppressant that acts in the brain, by contrast only costs $14/month.

Dietary Supplements:

Corey Ander came to see me because she had tried multiple diets and couldn't lose weight. She was middle-aged and had a time-consuming career as a plastic surgeon. Her BMI was high at 28. Due to her intense focus on her career, she did not exercise. Corey had an additional problem, however. She had developed a tremor.

When Corey came to my office, she was very upset. She had just finished a tummy tuck on a graduate student in negotiations and had shaken throughout the entire procedure. She was worried because a tremor could mean the end of her career. The first thing we did after obtaining routine laboratory work was to review her medications. There was nothing that would cause jitteriness, but the Metoprolol she was taking for high blood pressure and the antihistamine she was taking for her allergies could be contributing to her difficulty in losing weight.

We changed the blood pressure medication to Lisinopril and I took her off the antihistamine and put her on daily nasal saline rinses. After carefully reviewing her medical history, doing a physical, and obtaining the appropriate lab work, I still couldn't find the cause for her tremor. I decided to ask for more details.

"Corey, have you been taking any vitamins or supplements?"

"Nothing except raspberry ketones to help with my weight," she replied.

"There are no studies to support a role for raspberry ketones in weight loss and they could possibly cause jitteriness (Haslan and James 2005, 1197–1209). Why don't you try stopping them?"

She was flying out that afternoon for a week-long medical conference and would have time to get the raspberry ketones out of her system before returning to the OR after her conference.

After changing her medications, stopping the herbal supplement, and writing her an exercise prescription, I saw Corey again in a month. She had stopped shaking and had lost weight.

Even though the Food and Drug Administration regulates dietary supplements, it does not regulate them tightly and treats them like food. Unlike the manufactures of pharmaceuticals, herbal supplement producers do not have to have their products undergo studies to show they are safe and effective before putting them on the market.

Herbs, just because they are derived from natural plant sources, are not necessarily healthy. They can be very toxic. For instance, on April 12, 2004, the FDA banned the sale of products containing the herb ephedra, a weight-loss supplement. The reason was heart attacks, arrhythmias, strokes, psychosis, seizures, and death. Aristolochia is a Chinese herb included in weight loss herbal formulas and has been associated with over a hundred cases of renal disease. It also probably contributes to the development of cancer in the urogenital tract for those who take it. Besides cardiovascular and kidney problems, herbal supplements can cause interactions with medications that you may be taking.

Herbal supplements for weight loss are purported to work in about six different ways. Some increase energy expenditure. Others modulate carbohydrate metabolism or act through increasing satiety. Some claim to increase fat oxidation or reduce fat synthesis. Increasing water elimination or blocking dietary fat absorption are two other mechanisms of weight reduction.

Two of the herbs that fit into the energy expenditure category are ephedra (or ma huang) and bitter orange. They were found, when combined with caffeine, to be effective in modest weight loss. However, they have potentially serious or even lethal consequences. Raspberry ketones, a relatively new kid on the block, also works by increasing the burning of calories. This supplement has not been studied enough to demonstrate effectiveness or if it has similar potential side effects as the other herbs that exhibit their effectiveness in this manner.

Chromium, thought to modulate carbohydrate metabolism and to be useful in diabetics, has been shown to cause destruction of muscle and also to precipitate kidney failure. Ginseng is another herb that may improve sugar regulation. No studies have shown greater weight loss with ginseng than with placebo (Saper et al. 2004, 1731-1738).

Fiber weight-loss products increase satiety. These include glucomannan, psyllium, and guar gum. Glucomannan may help with modest weight loss, but the trials that concluded this were small and poorly designed (Saper et al. 2004, 1731-1738).   Guar gum and psyllium have no effect on weight loss, although psyllium improves glucose and cholesterol parameters.

Hydroxycitric acid (HCA), from the Malabar tamarind tropical fruit, is claimed to decrease fat synthesis, and it is the ingredient in garcinia cambosia. Evidence for this is contradictory, although the herb appears to be well tolerated. Conjugated linoleic acid is another supplement in this class, but it has been reported to cause gastrointestinal symptoms and there is no data to support its effectiveness in weight loss.

The weight-loss benefits of green tea, thought to increase fat oxidation and thermogenesis, were based on a study of only ten patients (Saper et al. 2004, 1731-1738) and the study wasn't looking at weight loss. Licorice, like green tea, has had success in the weight-loss department, but can cause hypertension and low potassium.

In the class of supplements that block fat absorption is chitosan. It appears to be safe in short-term studies, but the bulk of evidence shows that it is likely ineffective for weight loss. Dandelion and cascara are herbal supplements that work as a diuretic and laxative respectively. They can cause the same unwanted side effects as diuretics and laxatives in terms of electrolyte imbalance (Saper et al. 2004, 1731–1738).

Two popular weight-loss supplements are HCG and Vitamin B12, both given as injections. HCG is human chorionic gonadotropin hormone. It is produced by the placenta in pregnant women. HCG can also be produced by tumors of the ovaries and gonads. People who receive injections are receiving hormones derived from the urine of a pregnant woman. There is no scientific evidence to support the effectiveness of this protein in weight loss. In fact, the 500-calorie diet that accompanies the injections, is responsible for the weight loss. This is a dangerously low amount of calories. You should only undertake a very-low-calorie diet such as this under the supervision of a physician.

Vitamin B12 is also in vogue as a weight-loss enhancement. Like HCG, there is no scientific evidence to support a role for this supplement in weight loss. The use of B12 is based on the possibility that it will give its recipient more energy. However, that will only occur if one is deficient in this vitamin. Vitamin B12 deficiency is rare in people under sixty years old but can occur in vegetarians. An inexpensive blood test can be done to determine if you are B12 deficient. Even if your level is low, replacing it will not cause weight loss.

Sugar Substitutes:

Another addition to the weight-loss scene that you should be knowledgeable about are the sugar substitutes. There are two types: sugar alcohols and the artificial sweeteners. These are not the same. Sugar alcohols contain about 2.6 calories per gram and artificial sweeteners contain 0 calories (sugar contains 4 calories/gram). Sugar alcohols are about 50 to 70 percent as sweet as sugar and can contain a significant amount of carbohydrates. You should check the nutrition facts on the panel of the food to see the carbohydrate content. Artificial sweeteners contain no carbohydrates and are two hundred times as sweet as sugar.

The most common sugar alcohols are mannitol, sorbitol, xylitol, lactitol, isomalt, maltitol, and hydrogenated starch hydrolysates. These are all used in many foods we commonly consume, such as sugar-free gum and candies, sugar-free ice cream, chocolate, baked goods, cough drops, mouthwashes, and sugar-reduced preserves. The most common artificial sweeteners are saccharin (Sweet & Low) and aspartame (Equal or Nutrasweet).

Sugar alcohols can have side effects. Bloating and diarrhea occur when they are eaten in excessive amounts. Some people have these symptoms from a single serving. They can also cause a "laxative effect" and even cause weight gain when eaten in excess.

VI

Bariatric Medicine and Bariatric Surgery

Boe Wing came to me to lose weight and improve his health. He was fifty-seven years old and had a lot of life to live. Having had a thirty-year career as an airline pilot, he had flown hundreds of thousands of passengers safely to their destinations. Now his blood sugar and cholesterol were high, a consequence of his weight. He was concerned because he had had an episode of chest pain on a recent flight. Fortunately, there was a plastic surgeon on board heading to a medical conference. She was able to assess his chest discomfort and reassure him it was not cardiac, but also warned him that he was at risk for heart disease due to his weight. Now he was afraid that he would not pass his flight physical and would lose his job.

This pilot had a problem: an insatiable sweet tooth. His weight had seesawed over the years, and he had tried multiple different diets and even appetite-suppressing medications. At the time of his office visit, he weighed 278 pounds and his BMI was 37. His waist measurement was 45 inches (normal is less than forty for a man and less than thirty-five for a woman). Waist-to-hip ratio, which is even more important, should be less than 1 in a man and less than 0.8 in a woman (Jacobs et al. 2010, 1293–1301) and Boe's waist to hip ratio was high at 1.5. Boe played golf but rode in a cart and did not exercise regularly. He was at risk for a myocardial infarction.

My eyes sparkled with excitement when I met him and heard his history. I knew I could help him achieve his goal if he wanted to lose weight and avoid the kind of catastrophe that could result when a pilot has a heart attack in midflight.

"I am wondering if I really need to lose weight," he said.

"What?" I could not believe my ears.

"I've read about the obesity paradox," he continued. "Overweight people with coronary artery disease live longer than normal weight people with heart disease. Can you give me a note that says this so I can take it to my flight physical in case they don't want to pass me?"

"You have not read the recent literature," I said. "Purposeful weight loss is beneficial in people with coronary artery disease who are overweight. When weight loss is unintentional, as it was in the data that generated the conclusions you're familiar with, then coronary artery disease has a worse prognosis (Pack et al. 2014, 1368–1377). There is still speculation, however, about the obesity paradox. You need to shed the pounds and keep them off. You are at risk for diabetes and heart disease. The candy binges have got to go. "

He came to me because I am a bariatric physician, or in other words, an obesity medicine physician. I have expertise in the treatment of obesity and the genetic, biologic, environmental, social, and behavioral factors that contribute to being overweight. Methods that I employ for treatment include diet, physical activity recommendations, behavioral changes, meal substitutes (such as the ones I prescribed for Kara Mel), and pharmacotherapy.

Practicing this type of medicine often requires the assistance of other resources such as nutritionists, exercise physiologists, psychologists, and bariatric surgeons to optimize a healthy outcome for our patients. I know when it's appropriate to refer a patient for bariatric surgery, and Boe was a good candidate. Since he had failed conservative weight loss attempts for years as well as medical treatment with phentermine, this was the best solution for the pilot. Qualifying with a BMI of 37 and two comorbid conditions, which in his case were high blood sugar and high cholesterol, he was a good candidate. People who have a BMI of 40 or greater can be considered for weight reduction surgery, even if they don't have a comorbid condition. People with a BMI of less than 40 and greater than 35 who have a comorbid condition may be candidates for bariatric surgery.

Weight-loss surgery is associated with mortality (death) reduction (Buchwald et al. 2004, 1724–37). One of the most significant effects of weight-loss surgery is on diabetes with an 82 percent resolution at one year in a study of eighteen patients (Sjostrom et al. 2007, 741–752). The exact mechanism that is responsible for this phenomenon is still unknown.

In order to undergo the procedure, Boe would have to be screened to make sure he didn't have an endocrine disorder causing his weight problem. He would also have to be screened for depression, substance abuse, or an eating disorder. He would need to demonstrate that, once he had the surgery, he could follow a diet and would be willing to exercise.

There are four primary types of procedures available: the laparoscopic adjustable gastric band, the sleeve gastrectomy, the gastric bypass, and the duodenal switch. The laparoscopic adjustable gastric band is a surgery in which a band is placed around the entrance to the stomach. The surgery takes less than one hour and can be done as an outpatient or overnight. Recovery takes two weeks. It has the lowest mortality and complication rate out of the four surgeries. It also has a low malnutrition risk. On the downside, the laparoscopic adjustable gastric band surgery has the lowest success of the weight-loss surgeries. People lose 45 to 50 percent of excess body weight. Long term, however, 40 percent regain most of their weight.

The sleeve gastrectomy is the most common procedure performed in the United States today, and for good reason. The surgery takes only approximately one hour. It requires a one- or two-day hospital stay, and in two to three weeks, you can expect to be fully recovered. This procedure involves removing 75 to 80 percent of the stomach, making it about the size of a banana. Since nothing is bypassed, there is no malabsorption. Micronutrient deficiencies can occur, however, and you should be monitored for iron and copper deficiency. The surgery also takes away the hormone ghrelin, so you will feel less hungry. The sleeve gastrectomy surgery can be done laparoscopically. Patients can expect an average weight loss of 55% excess weight at three years.

Gastric bypass is a surgery in which the stomach is bypassed from the pylorus, or entrance, to the small intestine. It takes approximately one hour and forty minutes to perform the procedure. Hospital stay is about one to three days and full recovery is in four to six weeks. As evidenced by the fact that at ten years 60 to 70 percent of patients lost at least 50 percent of their excess body weight and kept it off, this surgery is effective for maintaining long-term weight control.

The duodenal switch is the most radical of the weight-loss surgeries and is reserved for the most severely weight challenged people. It is a malabsorption procedure and bypasses 80 to 90 percent of the small bowel. It is not commonly performed because a high fat malabsorption, with all the trimmings (such as chronic foul-smelling diarrhea) can accompany this outcome. About 80 percent of excess body weight is lost and remains gone after ten years.

As with any surgery, complications are possible with these procedures. Many of the complications are related to the particular type of weight-loss surgery. For example, the gastric band may slip. Or you may develop a gastric or intestinal leak if you've had a gastric bypass. Other risks include developing a bowel obstruction or stricture in which food can't pass through your GI tract.

Following a weight-loss surgery, you will have to be on a liquid diet for two weeks, then a pureed diet for two to four weeks, and finally transition to "real food" over the next four to eight weeks. You must embrace a new model for weight control in which you eat smaller portions, refrain from excessive snacking, eliminate sugary foods and soft drinks, take vitamins, and exercise.

A device from 1985 has re-emerged on the weight loss scene. It is the gastric balloon. Used in conjunction with a long-term supervised diet and behavior modification program, this modality can help you lose three times more weight over a 6 month period than with diet and exercise alone. The device is a soft silicone balloon that is inserted endoscopically and then inflated with saline fluid. The procedure takes 20 - 30 minutes as an outpatient. After 6 months, the balloon is punctured with a needle that is inserted endoscopically. The balloon is then grabbed with a wire grasper and extracted up the esophagus. Another type of balloon is encapsulated and is swallowed at an office visit. It is filled with saline through a catheter and gradually dissolves over a few months then passes into the toilet. Nausea and vomiting occur in most people for 2 weeks after insertion of this device (is this why they lose weight?). Abdominal pain and reflux are common. The cost is expensive and ranges between $4,000 - $10,000.

The AspirateAssist involves a simple outpatient procedure that is done in approximately 10 minutes that promises an average of 46 pounds of weight loss in the first year. A tube is inserted through the abdominal wall and into the stomach. After consuming a meal, you aspirate approximate 30% of the food you ate from your stomach and dump it into the toilet. Need I say more.

Weight-loss surgery is no picnic, but Boe flew through it. Six months after his gastric sleeve procedure, he had lost 50 pounds, which was approximately 60 percent of his excess body weight. In addition, he no longer had high blood sugar or high cholesterol and passed his flight physical.

VII

Habits

Otto DuWhitt worked at the fish counter in the local grocery store. Every day when he came to work, he would make a brief visit to the sausage department next door. His best friend was the sausage maker. Otto would have a breakfast of sausage donated by his friend and fresh biscuits donated by the admiring ladies in the bakery. Life was good until Otto noticed that he had gained 20 pounds. Trying to lose it, he went on a calorie-restricted diet but found he could not give up the morning sausage and biscuit breakfast. Otto came to me for help in changing his eating habits.

One of the most important aspects of weight management lies in eating habits. Once you decide to lose weight, where do you go to restructure your ingrained eating patterns? According to Charles Duhigg in his book The Power of Habit, a habit consists of a cue, a routine, and a reward. Habits are driven by cravings. Studies have shown that cravings occur when one repetitively experiences a cue, performs a routine, and achieves a reward. If the craving isn't satisfied, we can feel disappointed, angry or depressed (Duhigg 2012). That is why it is so hard to change habits.

If one were to use this model for healthy eating, one could see a scheduled eating time on the clock as the cue, eat a well-planned meal as the routine, and have a sense of satiation and healthy weight as the reward. The craving would be satisfied because you had developed a routine through repeating the same action, which resulted in a reward. However, this ideal scenario is not frequently the reality. You can't change your eating habits without knowing what are your cues, routines, and rewards. You may find, for example, that your reward is not satiation but rather is relief from boredom or fatigue. Perhaps your reward is comfort from loneliness, sadness, anger or stress. Identifying the reward is not always easy.

Once you have recognized the reward, you may be able to change the routine to achieve your goal. Instead of seeking out a doughnut to comfort your emptiness, you may be able to walk around the block or go to the gym and workout with other people (some of whom are likely there also to avoid the doughnut).

The routine is the behavior you want to change (Duhigg 2012). In the story of Otto DuWhitt, you may think the reward is the sausage biscuit. However, for Otto, the real reward was that he wanted a jump-start to his day and he loved the attention he received from the ladies in the bakery. Once he was able to identify this, he decided to go over to the bakery and chat with his flirtatious friends, and then return to work without consuming a 700-calorie sausage biscuit. His weight diminished and the attention from the bakery babes increased.

Otto realized that he needed a good habit. For a good habit to form, one needs to find another way to satisfy the craving through changing the routine. As I mentioned, you must have a cue, a routine, and a reward. When your brain starts expecting the reward with the new routine in place, a new habit will become established (Duhigg 2012). As a simplistic example, if you want to develop healthy eating habits, identify your cue with a clock that indicates a designated eating time. Then establish the routine of eating a healthy meal you enjoy. Your reward will be satiation and a sense of accomplishment for eating well. Further benefits will be better health, increased self-esteem, and an overall sense of feeling better.

But in order to achieve these important results, you must modify your old habit, as Otto did. You must repeat your new routine over and over until a craving forms. He knew that the cue was arriving at work and smelling the delicious aromas coming from the bakery. He liked a little jump-start to his day before settling into his work. As with most habits, the cue was not going to change. The bakery had to function and Otto was not going to get a new job. Once he figured out his true reward, which was jump-starting his day with the social satisfaction he got from visiting with the ladies in the bakery, he was able to change his routine. Instead of picking up a biscuit and going back to his friend's station to add some sausage and mustard, he took a cup of coffee over to the bakery and chatted with the bakery babes for a few minutes before starting his work. His cue did not change and his reward did not change. However, he was able to modify his routine and therefore achieve his weight goals.

When Otto came back to me for his six-month follow-up, he told me that he also had been attending a weekly weight-management group session sponsored by his local hospital. I praised him for his decision to do this, because people who attend groups for weight loss are more successful at losing weight and keeping it off than those who lose weight individually (Foreyt 2004, 1-3).

He also told me that his weight loss had helped resolve his back problems. He had just managed to haul 100 pounds of lobster ordered for the wedding of a pilot and plastic surgeon to a reception hall without any back pain. Otto was very pleased with his new habit.

VIII

The Rules of Eating

The National Weight Control Registry is evidence of the successful rules of weight management habits that work. It is a study of 10,000 individuals (eighteen years old or older) who have lost an average of 30 pounds each and have kept it for at least five and a half years. Only 4 percent in this study lost weight with the use of medication. The habits that worked included:

1. 98 percent have modified their food intake with portion control
2. 90 percent exercise on average over one hour per day, burning 400 calories
3. 78 percent eat breakfast every day
4. 75 percent weigh themselves once weekly
5. 62 percent watch less than ten hours of television a week

The women in the registry consume an average of 1,306 calories/day and the men take in an average of 1,685 calories/day (Graham et al. 2011, S1-S262).

I base my Rules of Eating and Weight Management on these findings as well as the information described so far in this book.

Rules of Eating and Weight Management

1. **PORTION CONTROL**. Use a sandwich plate instead of a dinner plate. No serving of a high-density food should be bigger than the palm of your hand. High-density foods include meats/proteins and legumes.

   Simple carbohydrates should be limited to none or very small portions.

2. **MAKE SURE TO EAT VERY SLOWLY**. It takes ten to twenty minutes for the brain to register that you've eaten and for a feeling of satiation to occur. Chew slowly. Put your fork down. Talk to someone. Hold your fork in your nondominant hand and use this hand for eating.

3. **EXERCISE**. Exercise daily and take advantage of the opportunity to engage in NEAT activities. Walk at work, take the stairs, stand rather than sit, fidget, and keep moving. Exercise and NEAT need to be priorities. If you need to, you should manipulate your other activities to fit in physical activity. It is that important!

4. **WEIGH YOURSELF DAILY OR AT LEAST WEEKLY**.
   You will find it easier to modify your food intake in terms of type of food and quantity when you see it reflected in your weight.

5. **COUNT YOUR CALORIES**. It's important to do this at least until you get in the habit of consuming a structured daily caloric goal. Remember: calories in = calories out. If you are consuming more calories than you are burning, you will gain weight. If you are taking in less, you will lose weight. Don't cheat yourself by forgetting that age, gender, and genetics enter into your daily caloric needs. Calculate those factors, along with exercise and activity, into your daily caloric plan. You will be rewarded! Caloric intake is the most important factor in weight loss.

6. **RESPECT YOUR ANCESTRY**. Your prehistoric family insured that your metabolism will slow down when you lose weight. Be

persistent and stick to your diet. Recalculate your caloric need every month as you lose weight.

7. **SPREAD YOUR CALORIC INTAKE OVER THE DAY**. Three meals and two or three snacks are a very tolerable way to manage hunger. Your weight-related hormones will thank you.

8. **UNDERSTAND YOUR EATING HABITS**. If you are not able to conform to a healthy eating cycle—which would be eating at a time-oriented cue, eating a healthy meal or snack, and feeling the reward of satiation and good health—then search for how you can make modifications or get help. Make an appointment with a bariatrician or your doctor for support and advice.

9. **DESIGN OR FOLLOW A DIET THAT YOU ENJOY**.

    Make it an enhancement to your life. We are all different and have different tastes. Many weight-loss programs are available and, as research has shown, one is not superior over another for weight loss and maintenance.

    Choose an eating plan that you enjoy.

    JUST REMEMBER: CALORIES IN = CALORIES OUT.

10. **THERE ARE NO MAGIC BULLETS**. Avoid herbs and weight-loss remedies that promise results that have not been verified through medical studies. A bariatric physician may be able to prescribe a safe and effective weight reducing medication, but this is only a temporary adjunct to following a structured food plan and exercise.

11. **BE CAREFUL ABOUT TAKING MEDICATIONS THAT MAY CAUSE WEIGHT GAIN**. You should talk to your doctor if you think you may be on weight-unfriendly medications.

12. **AIM FOR SLOW WEIGHT LOSS**. The most successful weight loss through dieting is slow weight loss with a 5 percent decrease over three months.

13. **GET ADEQUATE SLEEP.** There is a strong association between habitual sleep duration and weight. Moderate sleep duration of 7 to 8 hours each night leads to successful weight management.

14. **TALK TO A BARIATRIC PHYSICIAN**. If you need extra help or are considering weight loss surgery, consult a bariatric physician. You may find a bariatric physician through the Obesity Society (http://www.obesity.org).

The Doctor's Diet

As we know, our bodies are still wired with the prehistoric metabolism that evolved when weight gain was a survival mechanism. The Doctor's Diet works because it helps convince the body that it doesn't need to accumulate fat for the cold winter of starvation ahead. Essential to the diet are limiting portion size (so the body doesn't think it's hoarding food) and eating small amounts consistently throughout the day to avoid significant hunger (so the body doesn't think it's starving). Exercise is critical because the body needs to know we are hunting and gathering, and not preparing for hibernation. This eating program includes probiotics and prebiotics which help promote healthy gut flora for efficient digestion. It is high in fiber and complex carbohydrates. These foods are digested slowly and help satiation so one doesn't reach for another serving with each meal. The Doctor's Diet has two servings of protein, another food group that provides appetite satisfaction. Also included in the diet are fats. Fats are essential for the absorption of vitamins and they support cell growth. Most importantly, this diet includes treats, the foods you love! It is simple, flexible, and fun so you can stick to it for a lifetime.

THE DIET: 1400 calories
(Calories can be adjusted in the non-treat foods depending upon your needs)

- Two 150 gram servings of low fat yogurt (100 calories each)
- Two servings of lean protein
- Three to four servings of prebiotics/complex carbohydrates that are not legumes

- One ounce of cheese with five thin crackers (water crackers are a good choice)
- Two treats that are less than or equal to 200 calories each
- Beverages: water, coffee, tea, red wine (calories with these must be counted as "treat" calories)

These foods should be spread out and consumed at no less than 5 to 6 intervals during the day with minimal hunger in between eating. No serving of protein should be bigger than the palm of your hand and complex carbohydrate servings should be about one cup each. A treat can be anything you love, as long as it's not over 200 calories.

If one is lactose intolerant, probiotic supplements can be added daily and a 100 calorie high fiber food can be substituted for each serving of yogurt.

Rules of Eating and Weight Management

- **PORTION CONTROL**
- **MAKE SURE TO EAT VERY SLOWLY**
- **EXERCISE**
- **WEIGH YOURSELF DAILY OR AT LEAST WEEKLY**
- **COUNT YOUR CALORIES**
- **RESPECT YOUR ANCESTRY**
- **UNDERSTAND YOUR EATING HABITS**
- **DESIGN OR FOLLOW A DIET THAT YOU ENJOY**
- **THERE ARE NO MAGIC BULLETS**
- **BE CAREFUL ABOUT TAKING MEDICATIONS THAT MAY CAUSE WEIGHT GAIN**
- **AIM FOR SLOW WEIGHT LOSS**
- **GET ADEQUATE SLEEP**
- **TALK TO A BARIATRIC PHYSICIAN**

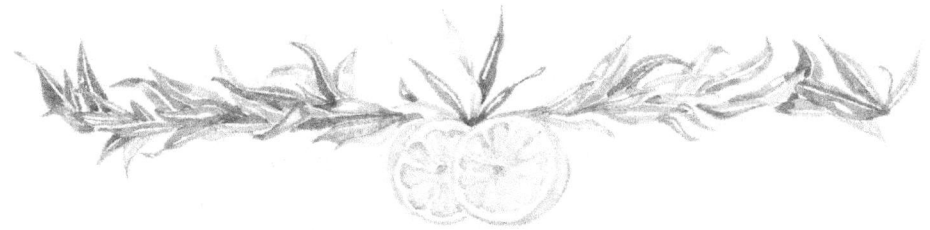

Conclusion

My daily trips to the grocery store usually bring pleasant surprises. This day was no exception. I ran into Conor Weezil at the bakery. He was admiring a wedding cake that was in the process of being frosted.

"Conor, you are looking as handsome as ever," I said.

"I know," he replied. "What do you think of my wedding cake?"

"You're getting married?" I asked. "Who's the lucky girl?"

"The fortunate woman is a gorgeous meteorologist for a national network. Her name is Kara Mel. I just finished negotiating our prenuptial agreement."

"I'm sure you've treated her fairly," I said.

"I will do very well if she ever decides to leave me," he proudly responded.

At that moment, Ellie popped her head out from behind the bakery counter.

"I like what you're doing with my wedding cake," said Conor.

"It's not yours," Ellie replied. "It's mine! And it's made with chickpeas!"

"Who are you marrying, Ellie?" I asked.

"Otto from the fish department," she said.

"Congratulations!" I said.

"Do you need a prenuptial agreement?" asked Conor Weezil.

I left Conor and Ellie alone to discuss wedding cakes and prenuptial agreements. I was pleased. My patients had succeeded in conquering their weight problems. After failed attempts with traditional diet methods, each found that weight loss and maintenance were achievable. Conor lost weight by recalculating his metabolic needs when he learned that metabolism slumps with weight loss through diet. Kara Mel lost her weight through a physician-supervised very-low-calorie diet.

Exercise was the solution that my middle-aged patient, Ellie, needed to keep her weight from increasing. By changing weight-unfriendly medications to weight-friendly medicines, Dr. Ander was able to diminish her struggle to lose weight. Boe Wing benefited from bariatric surgery. Habit changes were the key to success for Otto DuWhitt. *They all followed the Rules of Eating and a diet and exercise program that they enjoyed.*

My patients were able to lose weight and keep it off because they did it their "weigh."

So ended another trip to the local store.

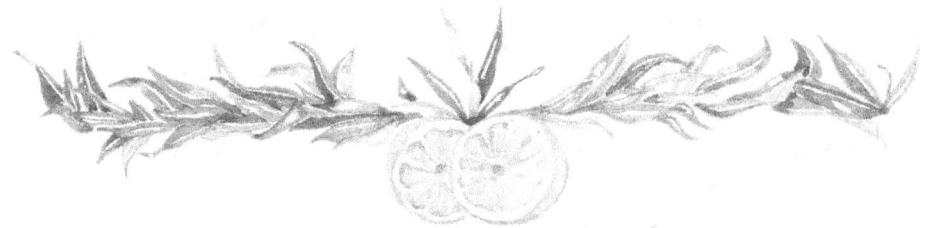

References

Alpert, JS. 2011. "You only have to exercise on the days that you eat." American Journal of Medicine124: 1.

Bassik S, Manson J. 2005. "Epidemiological Evidence for the Role of Physical Activity in Reducing the Risk of Type 2 Diabetes and Cardiovascular Disease." Journal of Applied Physiology 99: 1193–1204.

Bays HE. 2009. "Lorcaserin and adiposopathy: 5 HTZC agonism as a treatment for 'sick fat' and metabolic disease." Expert Review of Cardiovascular Therapy 7: 1429–1445.

Bazzano, Hu, Reynolds, Yao, Bunol, Liu, et al. 2014. "Effects of low-carbohydrate and low-fat diets. A randomized trial." Annals of Internal Medicine 161.5: 309–318.

Boden W, Franklin B, Berra K, et al. 2014. "Exercise as a therapeutic intervention in patients with stable ischemic heart disease: an underfilled prescription." American Journal of Medicine. 127.10: 905–911.

Bosquet L, Merkari S, Arvisais D, Aubert AE. 2008. "Is heart rate a convenient tool to monitor over-reaching? A systematic review of the literature." British Journal of Sports Medicine 42: 709.

Bray GA, and C Bouchard. 2008. Handbook of Obesity. New York: Informa Healthcare.

Buchwald H, Avidor Y, Braunwald E, et al. 2004. "Bariatric surgery: a systemic review and meta-analysis." JAMA 292.14: 1724–37.

Chang J, Sangeta K. 2014. "The protein-sparing modified fast for obese patients with type 2 diabetes: what to expect." Cleveland Clinic Journal of Medicine 81.9: 557–565.

Di Baise JK, Frank DN, Mathur R. 2012. "Impact of the gut microbiota on the development of obesity: current concepts." American Journal of Gastroenterology supplement 1: 22–27.

Duhigg, C. 2012. The Power of Habit. New York: Random House.

Foreyt JP. 2004. "Weight loss: counseling and long-term management." Medscape Diabetes and Endocrinology 612: 1-3. Medscape Multispecialty. www.medscape.com/viewarticle/493028

Freedman MR, King J, Kennedy E. 2001. "Popular diets: a scientific review." Obesity Research 9.1: 1S-40S.

Gadde K, Allison D, Ryan D, et al. 2011. "Effects of low-dose, controlled release, phentermine plus topiramate combination on weight and associated comorbidities in overweight and obese adults (CONQUER): a randomized, placebo-controlled, phase 3 trial." Lancet 377.9774: 1341-1352.

Graham T, et al. 2011. "Ten-year weight change in the national weight control registry." Obesity 2011 Abstract Supplement 19.1: S1-S262. www.nwcr.ws.research.2011

Haslan DW, James WP. 2005. "Obesity." Lancet_366.9492: 1197–1209. WebMD. http://www.webmd.com/diet/raspberry-ketones-uses-risks

Heymsfield SB, JB Harp, ML Reitman ML, et al. 2007. "Why Do Obese Patients Not Lose More Weight When Treated with Low Calorie Diets? A Mechanistic Perspective." American Journal of Clinical Nutrition 85: 346.

Jacobs EJ, Newton CC, Wang Y, et al. 2010. "Waist circumference and all cause mortality in a large US cohort." Archives of Internal Medicine 170: 1293–1301.

Johnston BC, et al. 2014. "Comparison of weight loss among named diet programs in overweight and obese adults: a meta-analysis." JAMA 312.9: 923–933.

Kodama S, Saito K, Tanaka S, et al. 2009. "Cardiorespiratory fitness as a quantitative predictor of all cause mortality and cardiovascular events in healthy men and women: a meta-analysis." JAMA_301: 2024.

Koster A, Leitzmann MF, Schatzkin A, et al. 2008. "General and abdominal adiposity and risk of death in Europe." New England Journal of Medicine 359: 2105–2120.

Kushi LH, Doyle C, McCullough M, et al. 2012. "American Cancer Society Guidelines on nutrition and physical activity for cancer prevention; reducing the risk of cancer with healthy food choices and physical activity." CA: A Cancer Journal for Clinicians_62: 30.

Ladabaum U, Mannalithara A, Myer P, Singh G. 2014. "Obesity, abdominal obesity, physical activity, and caloric intake in US adults: 1988–2010." The Am J of Med 127.8: 717–727.

Leung Yinko, et al. 2014. "Fish consumption and acute coronary syndrome." The American Journal of Medicine 127.9: 848–857.

Medline Plus. 2015. Diets. http://www.nlm.nih.gov/medline plus/diets. html#cat1

Michaud DS, Giovannucci E, Willett WC, et al. 2001. "Physical activity, obesity, height and the risk of pancreatic cancer." JAMA_286: 921.

National Institute of Health, National Heart, Lung and Blood Institute. 2000. The practical guide: identification, evaluation, and treatment of overweight and obesity in adults. NIH Publication Number 00–4084. Washington, DC: GPO. http://www.nhlbi.nih.gov/guidelines/obesity/prctgs_c.pdf

Nordmann AJ, Nordmann A, Briel M, et al. 2013. "Effects of low-carbohydrate vs low fat diets on weight loss and cardiovascular risk factors: a meta-analysis of randomized controlled trials." Archives of Internal Medicine 166.3: 285–293.

Pack QR, Rodriguez-Excudero JP, Thomas R, et al. 2014. "The prognostic importance of weight loss in coronary artery disease: a systemic review and meta-analysis." Mayo Clinic Proceedings 89.10: 1368–1377.

Pate RR, Pratt M, Blair SN, et al. 1995. "Physical activity and public health. A recommendation from the Centers for Disease Control and Prevention and the American College of Sports Medicine." JAMA 273: 402.

Roberts SB, and I Rosenberg. 2006. "Nutrition and Aging: Changes in the Regulation of Energy Metabolism with Aging." Physiology Review 86: 651.

Rowe GC, Safdar A, Arany Z. 2014. "Running forward: new frontiers in endurance exercise biology." Circulation 129: 798–810.

Saper R, Eisenberg D, Phillips R. 2004. "Common dietary supplements for weight loss." American Family Physician 70.9: 1731–1738.

Schwartz A, and E Doucet. 2010. "Relative Changes in Resting Energy Expenditure during Weight Loss: A Systemic Review." Obesity Review 11.7 (July): 531–547.

Sjostrom L, Narbro K, Sjostrom CD, et al. 2007. "Effects of bariatric surgery on mortality in Swedish obese subjects." New England Journal of Medicine 357.8: 741–752.

Sofi F, Cesari F, Abbate P, et al. 2008. "Adherence to Mediterranean diet and health status: meta-analysis." British Medical Journal 337: 1344.

Strasser B, Siebert U, Schobersberger W. 2010. "Resistance training in the treatment of the metabolic syndrome: a systematic review and meta-analysis of the effect of resistance training on metabolic clustering in patients with normal glucose metabolism." Sports Medicine 40: 397.

Sumithran P, LA Prendergast, E Delbridge E, et al. 2011. "Long-Term Persistence of Hormonal Adaptations to Weight Loss." New England Journal of Medicine 365: 1597-1604.

Tooze JA, DA Schoeller, AF Subar, et al. 2007. "Total Daily Energy Expenditure among Middle-Aged Men and Women: The OPEN Study." American Journal of Clinical Nutrition 86: 382.

University of Vermont College of Medicine, et al. 2015. BMI chart,

Area health education centers program, www.uvm.edu

Villablanca P, et al. 2015. "Nonexercise activity thermogenesis in obesity management." Mayo Clinic Proceedings 90.4: 509–519.Wadden T, Neiberg R, Wing R, et al. 2011. "Four-Year Wight Losses in the Look AHEAD Study: Factors Associated with Long Term Success." NHPA Manuscript. http://www.ncbi.nlm.nih.gov/pmc/articles/pmc3183129/

Westerterp K. 2004. "Diet Induced Thermogenesis Review." Nutrition and Metabolism. 1–5.

Wisloff U, Ellingsen, Kemi OJ. 2009. "High-intensity interval training to maximize cardiac benefits of exercise training?" Exercise Sports Science Reviews Journal 37: 139.

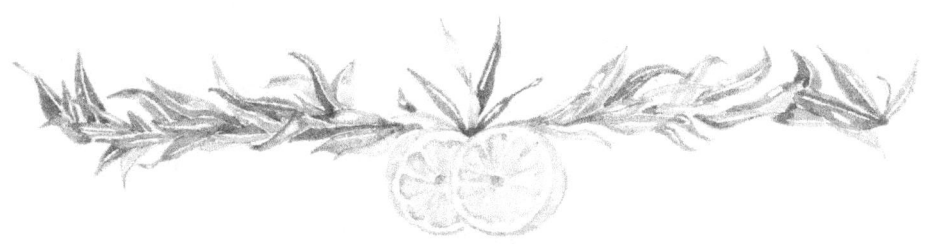

Part II
Recipes

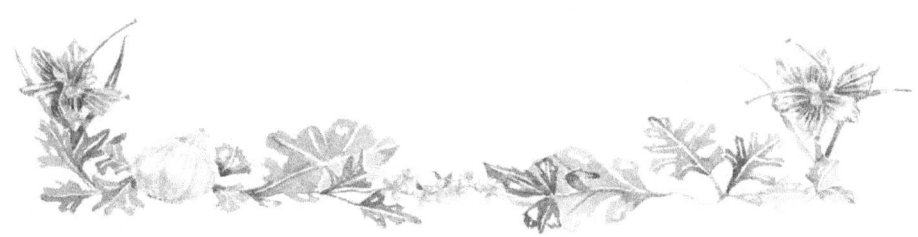

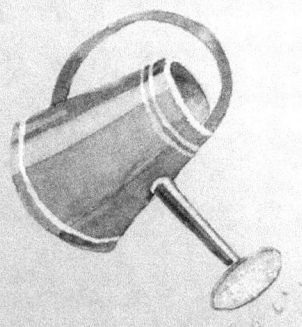

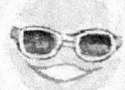

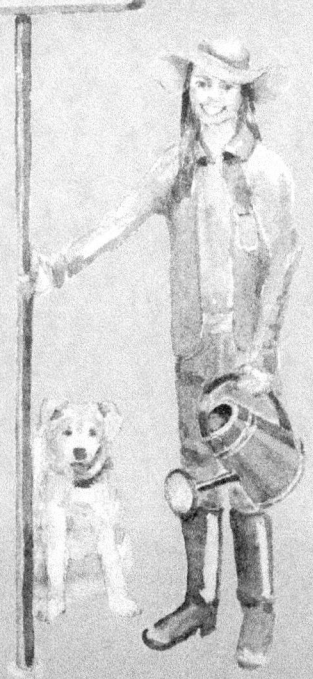

Sunshine Farms

LOCAL STORE SPECIALS

BOK CHOY

BROCCOLI

CAULIFLOWER

FENNEL

FISH

GREEN BEANS

GREENS

LEEKS

ONIONS

SQUASH

TOMATO

TURNIP

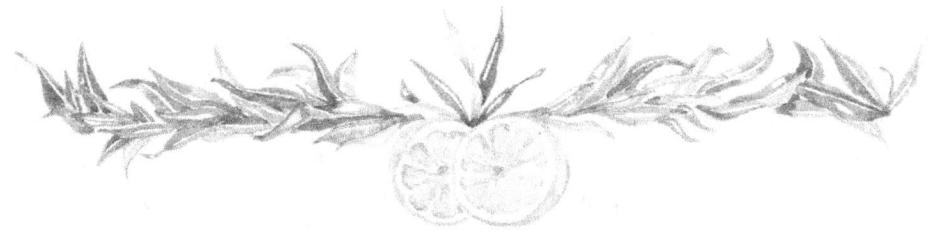

A Note from Dr. Cully Narrie:

Recipes for Weight Management and Good Health

The foods and recipes I have chosen for this book focus on vegetables and fish that will help you with your weight loss or weight maintenance. I have designed recipes that take advantage of the benefits of complex carbohydrates. In addition, most of the recipes include foods that are high in fiber. I use fresh, locally grown vegetables, and for an extra health kick, I use olive oil to pump up many of the recipes.

All of the dishes feature a main ingredient that is high in complex carbohydrates or protein. Complex carbohydrates and proteins are metabolized slower than simple carbohydrates (simple carbohydrates include breads, wheat products, rice, cakes, cookies, potatoes, soda and sweetened drinks, pasta, and sugary/sweet fruits). The complex carbohydrates and proteins are considered to have a low glycemic index. This means that they cause insulin to be secreted slowly and steadily. Insulin is the hormone that metabolizes the sugar in our blood and when insulin is secreted rapidly in response to a high glycemic index food (simple carbohydrate), it causes a sudden drop in blood sugar. After the drop in blood sugar, you will quickly feel hungry, eat more, and gain weight. Therefore, if you want to maintain or achieve a healthy weight, you will benefit by eating a diet high in complex carbohydrates and low in simple carbohydrates.

Although I have not included them in my recipes because they are generally high in calories, legumes are a wonderful source of complex carbohydrates. This food group includes beans, peas, and lentils. They are low in fat, are a good source of protein, and contain both soluble and insoluble fiber.

Fiber is an essential ingredient to healthy nutrition. The average fiber intake for adults and children, however, is less than half the recommended values of 14 grams/1,000 calories. People who eat high amounts of fiber are at significantly lower risk for developing obesity. They are also at lower risk for developing coronary artery disease, hypertension, diabetes, and stroke. Blood pressure and cholesterol are lowered by increased intake of fiber. Increasing soluble fiber in one's diet improves insulin sensitivity and therefore improves metabolism in people with or without diabetes. Fiber also helps with gastric reflux, duodenal ulcer, constipation, and diverticulitis.

There are two types of fiber: soluble and insoluble. Soluble fiber dissolves in water and is found in oats, peas, beans, carrots, barley, apples, oranges, and other citrus fruits. This type of fiber lowers cholesterol and increases insulin sensitivity. Insoluble fiber adds bulk to stool and helps with constipation. It is found in wheat flour, wheat bran, beans, and vegetables such as broccoli, cauliflower, and the root vegetables. Both types of fiber are important to have in one's diet.

I enjoy cooking with fresh locally grown organic produce. There are two reasons for this. The first is that organic produce is better for one's digestion. Many of our digestive woes can be attributed to foods that are laced with antibiotics, pesticides, and chemical fertilizers. Over time, these elements change the gut flora and make it difficult for us to digest and process fiber and nutrients. The result is abdominal discomfort, gas, and weight gain. The second reason why I prefer fresh local produce is that it has a higher nutritive value than foods that are imported from locations long distances away. Fruits and vegetables begin to lose their nutritional value as soon as they are picked. The longer produce sits before it is consumed, the more nutrition is lost. If it is locally grown, chances are it hasn't been in a truck or on the shelf for very long.

I use olive oil in much of my cooking. There are different types of olive oil, and one must be careful because, although mandated by laws in Europe, there is no law in the United States to regulate the "virginity" of olive oil. This is significant, as extra virgin olive oil offers greater health benefits than virgin or nonvirgin olive oil. Olive oil processed in the United States may or may not live up to its label.

In addition to benefiting the cardiovascular system and helping to reduce inflammation, olive oil may also help to control insulin. The mechanisms responsible for the effects of olive oil on insulin have not been fully elucidated, although there is evidence to suggest that lower weight gain and food and calorie intake are associated with olive oil consumption.

Sesame oil, which I use to enhance Asian flavors, also offers health benefits similar to olive oil. But even though very similar in caloric content (120 calories/tablespoon of sesame oil), it is only about half as rich in monounsaturated fat as is olive oil.

Enjoy!

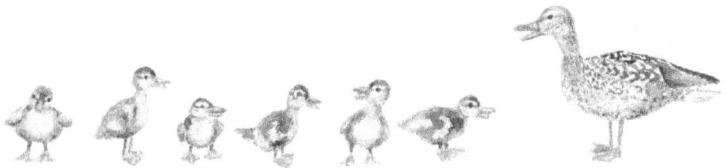

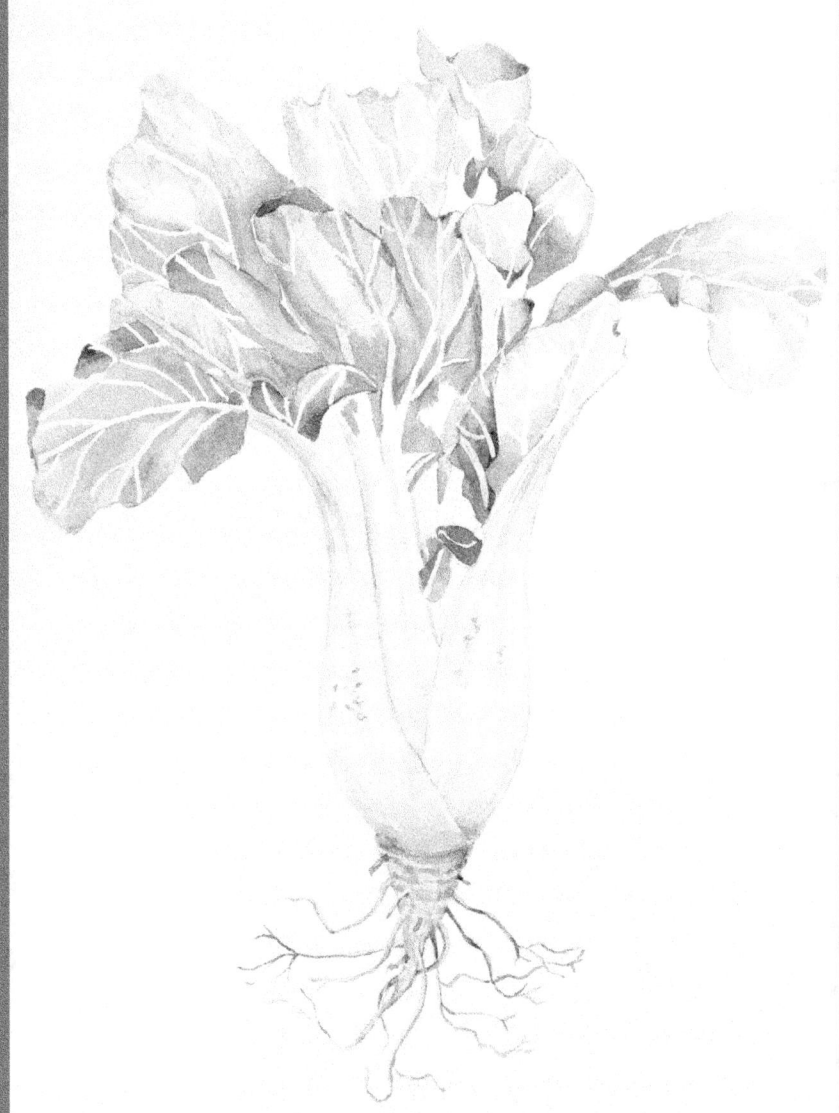

BOK CHOY

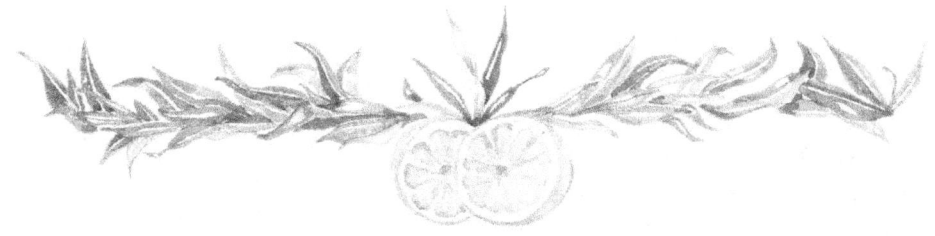

Recipes

Stir-Fry Bok Choy

- 3 garlic cloves, minced
- 1 teaspoon fresh ginger, grated
- 1 tablespoon olive oil
- ½ teaspoon salt
- 1 large bok choy, or 2 baby bok choy
- 3 tablespoons low-sodium chicken stock, water, or
- White wine
- Sesame oil

Mince garlic and grate ginger.
Add to a cold wok containing the oil.
Add salt.
Heat over medium-high heat until the garlic is golden and translucent.
Add bok choy.
Toss quickly for 15 to 20 seconds.
Add water, wine, or chicken stock.
Cover and cook 1 minute.

Drizzle with sesame oil.
Serve as side dish.

Servings: 2
Calories: 78 calories/serving

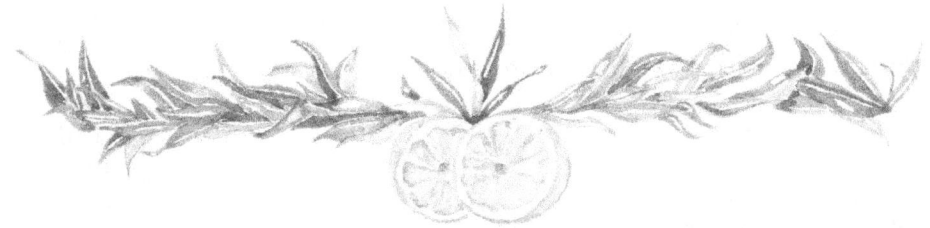

Bok-Choy Salad

- 2 cups thinly sliced bok choy
- ½ red pepper, sliced
- ½ cup carrots, shredded
- ½ cup fennel, thinly sliced
- ¼ cup green onions, sliced
- ¼ cup cilantro, chopped
- ¼ cup peanuts, chopped

Dressing:

- 1 tablespoon soy sauce
- 1 tablespoon brown sugar
- 2 teaspoons rice vinegar
- 2 teaspoons lime juice
- 1 garlic clove, minced
- 1 teaspoon fresh ginger, grated
- 1 teaspoon sesame oil
- 1 tablespoon olive oil

Toss vegetables.
Whisk together ingredients for dressing.
Add dressing as desired.

Servings: 6
Calories: 64 calories/serving

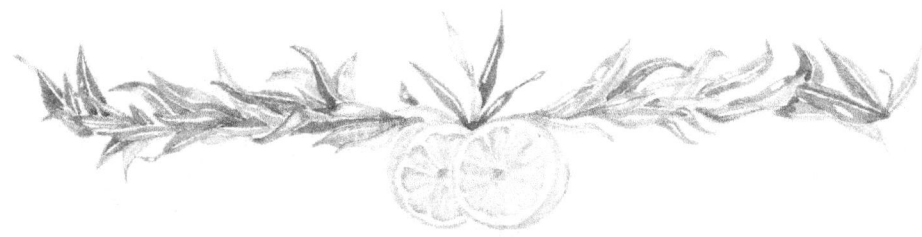

Bok Choy And Shrimp

- 3 garlic cloves, minced
- 1 teaspoon fresh ginger, grated
- 3 tablespoons shallots, minced
- 2 tablespoons olive oil
- ½ teaspoon salt
- 3 baby bok choy, leaves separated
- ½ pound shrimp (21 to 25), peeled and deveined
- 3 tablespoons low-sodium chicken stock or white wine

Mince garlic and grate ginger. Mince shallots.
Add to a cold wok containing olive oil. Add salt.
Heat over medium-high heat until garlic and shallots are translucent.
Add bok choy and shrimp, and toss for 15 seconds.
Add chicken stock or white wine.
Cover and cook until shrimp is pink, about 2 minutes.
Drizzle with sesame oil and zest with lemon rind.

Servings: 2
Calories: 166 calories/serving

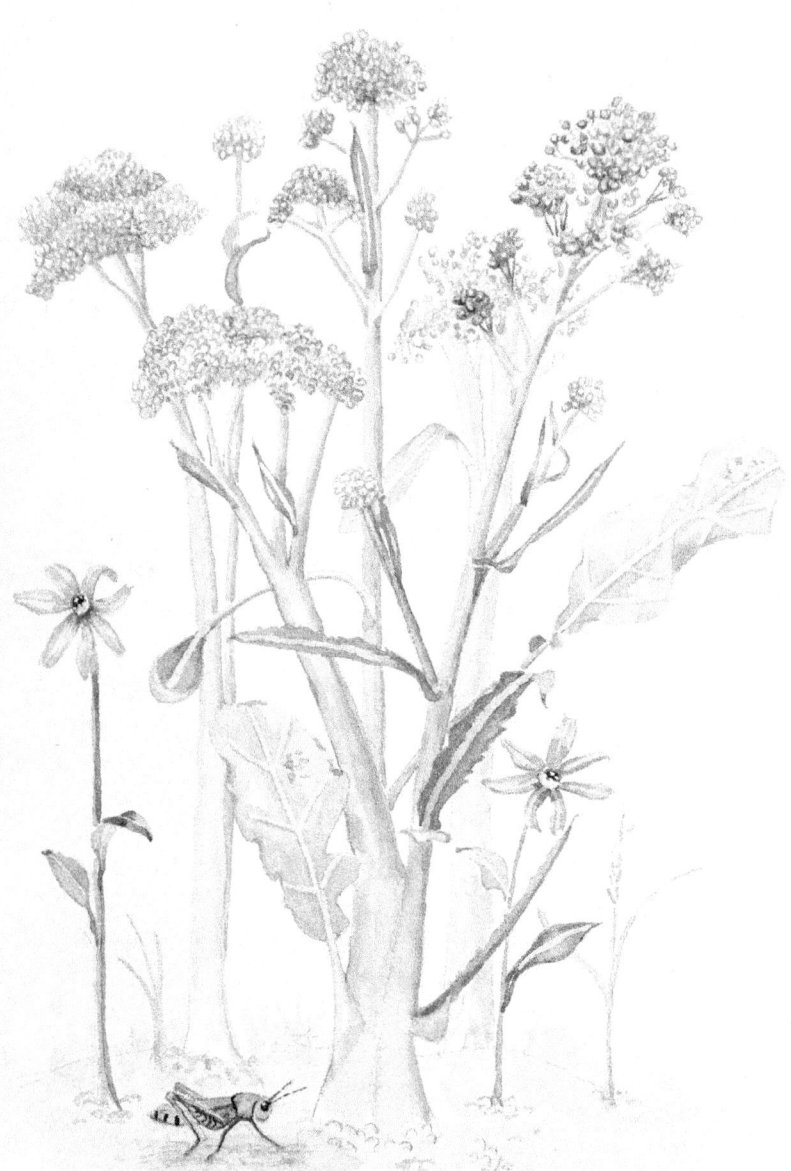

BROCCOLI

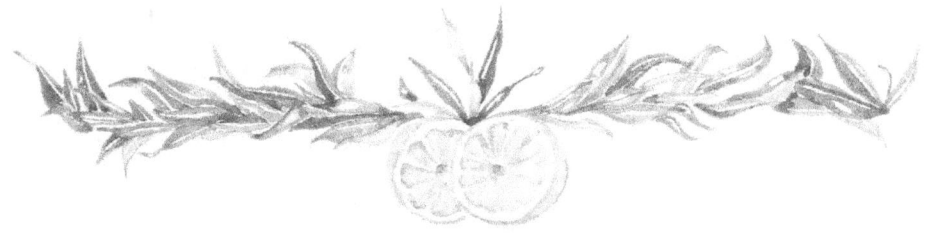

Roasted Broccoli

- 3 cloves garlic
- 2 tablespoons olive oil
- 1 tablespoon balsamic vinegar
- ¼ teaspoon salt and ⅛ teaspoon pepper
- 1 head broccoli (about 3 cups)

Preheat oven to 375 degrees.
Mince 3 cloves of garlic and soak in olive oil and balsamic vinegar.
Add salt and pepper.
Cut broccoli into florets. Toss in olive oil mixture.
Place on a baking sheet and cook for 20 minutes.

Servings: 4
Calories: 82 calories/serving

Sautéed Broccoli

- 6 cups water with 1 teaspoon salt
- 1 pound broccoli with stems
- 3 tablespoons olive oil
- 6 garlic cloves, minced
- ½ teaspoon salt

Cut bottom ¼ stems from broccoli and slice stalks lengthwise. Add to 6 cups boiling, salted water.
Cook for 2 minutes, drain, and immerse in ice water.
In a sauté pan, add olive oil and heat until glistening.
Add garlic and cook for 1 minute.
Add broccoli and salt, and sauté for 4 minutes.

Servings: 4
Calories: 119 calories/serving

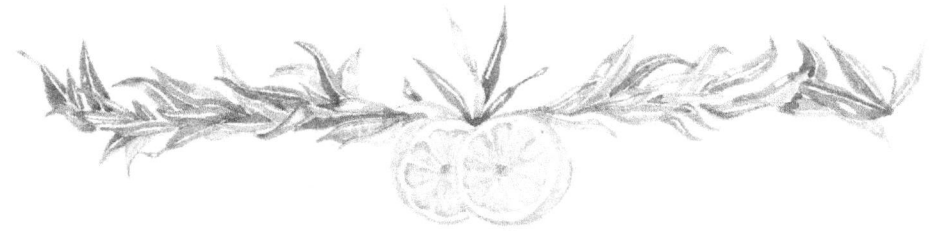

Broccolini and Orange Pieces

- ¼ cup almonds, chopped
- 1 orange, peeled and sections separated
- 1 tablespoon olive oil
- 3 garlic cloves, minced
- 1 bunch broccolini
- ⅓ cup water with ½ teaspoon salt
- ½ teaspoon smoked paprika
- 2 teaspoons sherry wine vinegar

In 425-degree oven, toast almonds and heat orange slices for about 5 minutes.

Heat olive oil in sauté pan; add garlic, and sauté for 1 minute. Add broccolini, salt, and sauté for 2 to 3 minutes until it begins to brown.

Add ⅓ cup water and cook for about 4 minutes (broccolini should still be crisp).

Cut cooked orange sections into ½-inch pieces.

Mix almonds, orange pieces, paprika, and vinegar, and pour over broccolini in a bowl. Toss and serve.

Servings: 4
Calories: 111 calories/serving

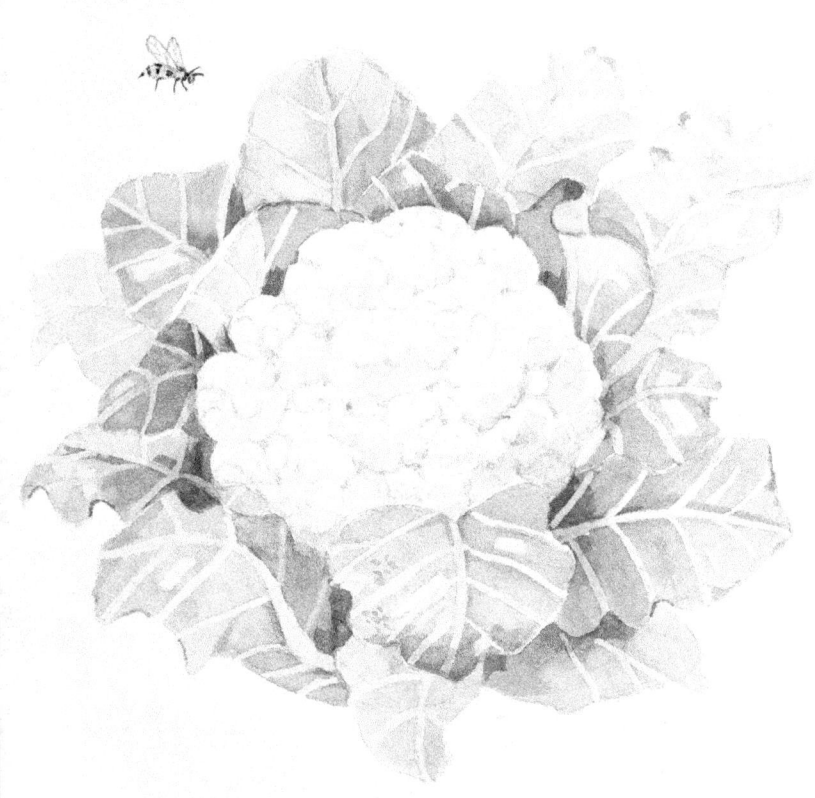

CAULIFLOWER

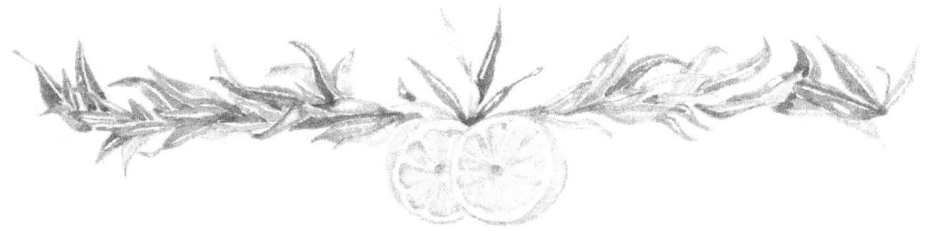

Roasted Cauliflower

- 2 cloves garlic, minced
- 2 tablespoons olive oil
- ½ teaspoon salt
- ¼ teaspoon black pepper
- ½ head cauliflower

Preheat oven to 425 degrees.
Combine garlic, olive oil, salt, and pepper, and soak at least 5 minutes.
Pull off leaves of cauliflower.
Cut around core and remove it.
Cut florets into 1-inch pieces.
Toss cauliflower pieces with olive oil/garlic/salt/pepper mixture.
Distribute coated pieces evenly on a piece of aluminum foil.
Cook at 425 degrees in middle of oven for 20 minutes or until slightly golden.

Servings: 4
Calories: 81 calories/serving

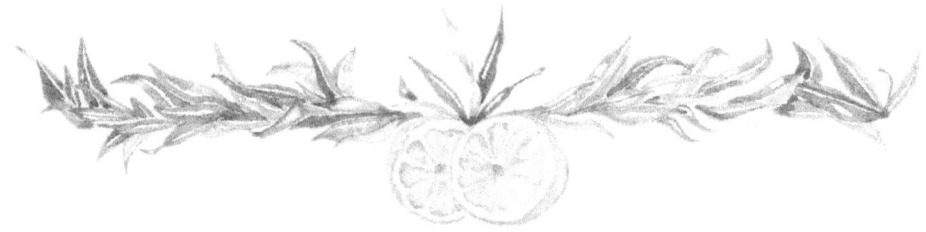

Cauliflower Soup

- 1 head cauliflower
- 2 tablespoons unsalted butter
- 1 leek, only white part, sliced thinly after cleaning and discarding dark green ends
- 1 medium white onion, sliced thinly
- 5 cups water
- ½ teaspoon salt
- ½ teaspoon curry
- ½ teaspoon sherry wine vinegar
- Almonds, toasted and chopped for garnish

Pull off leaves of cauliflower. Trim out core; slice into ½-inch pieces, and save. Slice florets into 1-inch pieces.

Melt butter in saucepan, and add leek, white onion, and salt. Cook until leeks and onions are translucent.

Add 5 cups water, salt, and half of sliced cauliflower, including core. Bring water to boil then reduce to simmer.

Simmer for 15 minutes.

Add rest of cauliflower and simmer another 20 minutes.

Process in a blender until smooth. Add curry and vinegar.

Return puree to pan and simmer over medium heat for about 3 minutes. Garnish with toasted chopped almonds.

Servings: 4
Calories: 172 calories/serving

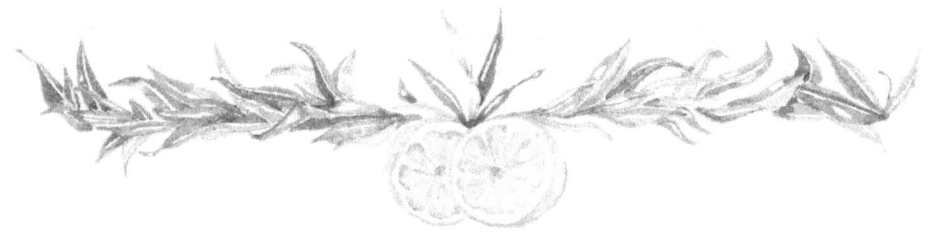

Cauliflower and Brussels Sprouts

- 1 tablespoon olive oil
- 2 cloves garlic, minced
- ½ head cauliflower, florets sliced
- ½ pound Brussels sprouts, sliced
- ½ red onion, sliced
- ½ teaspoon salt
- ½ cup water

Heat olive oil in a skillet.
Add garlic and sauté for a minute.
Add cauliflower, Brussels sprouts, onion, and salt.
Cook until vegetables just begin to brown.
Add water and cook until evaporated and vegetables are tender.

Servings: 4
Calories: 62 calories/serving

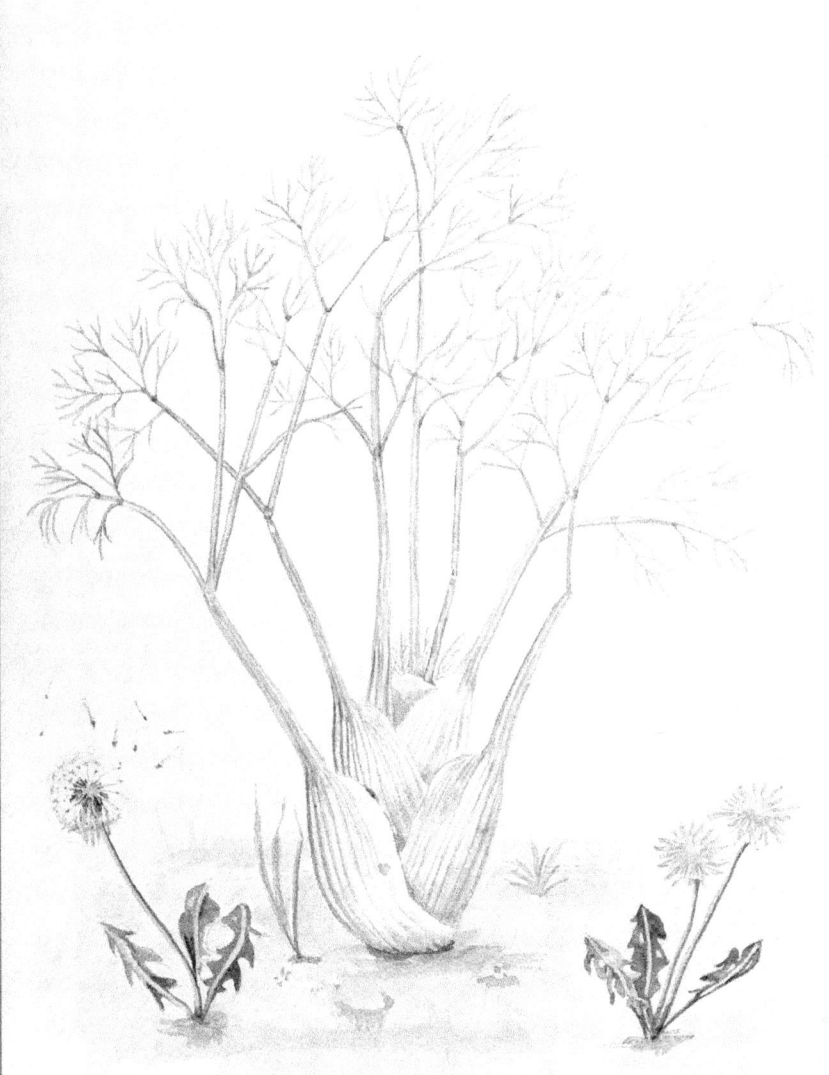

FENNEL

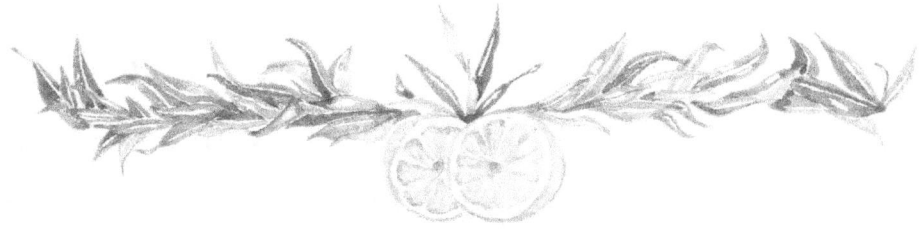

Braised Fennel

- 4 large fennel bulbs, sliced into ¼ inch slices
- 1 shallot, thinly sliced
- 1 cup low-sodium chicken stock
- ½ teaspoon salt
- ½ teaspoon pepper
- ¼ teaspoon ground nutmeg
- ¼ cup Panko bread crumbs
- ¼ cup shredded Parmesan cheese

Cut off roots and fronds of fennel bulbs.

Slice bulb lengthwise into ¼-inch slices.

Arrange fennel and shallot on the bottom of a baking dish.

Mix chicken stock, salt, pepper, and nutmeg, and pour over fennel.

Top with breadcrumbs and cheese.

Cover and bake for 20 minutes.

Remove cover and bake another 20 minutes or until fennel is tender.

Servings: 4
Calories: 106/serving

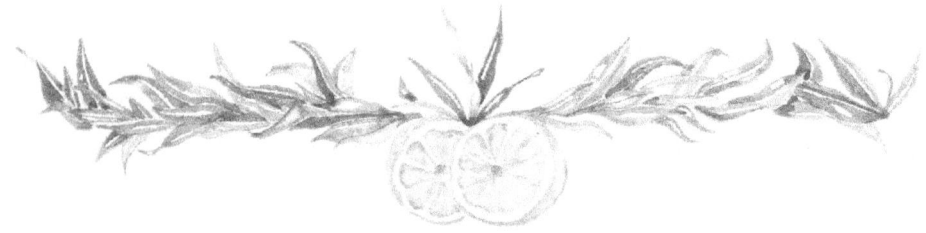

Roasted Fennel

- 4 fennel bulbs, sliced into ½-inch slices
- ½ teaspoon salt
- 2 tablespoons olive oil
- ¼ teaspoon ground red pepper
- 3 garlic cloves, minced
- 2 tablespoons Parmesan cheese

Preheat oven to 450 degrees.

In a bowl, combine fennel and remaining ingredients except cheese. Toss. Place fennel mixture in baking dish and cook at 450 degrees for 15 minutes.

During the last 2 minutes, sprinkle with Parmesan cheese.

Serving: 4
Calories: 118 calories/serving

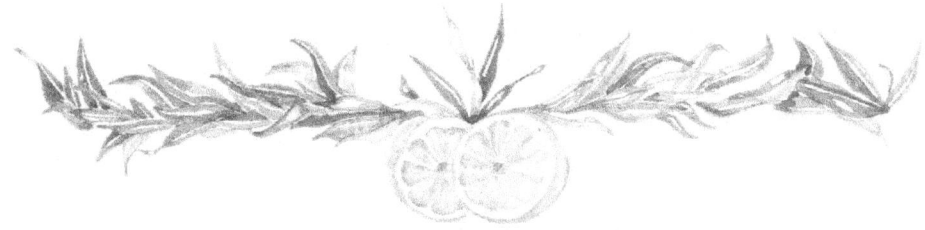

Green Bean and Fennel Salad

- ½ pound green beans, halved with ends cut off (about
- 2 cups)
- 3 cups water with ½ teaspoon salt
- ¼ cup sugar
- ⅓ cup red wine vinegar
- 1 tablespoon fresh basil, chopped
- 2 tablespoons olive oil
- Salt and pepper to taste
- 1 orange, peeled and segmented
- ½ red onion, thinly sliced
- ½ cup toasted pecans
- 2 medium fennel bulbs, thinly sliced lengthwise (about 3 cups)
- 8 ounces or about ½ pound mixed greens

Cook green beans in ½-inch boiling salted water in a skillet for 6 to 8 minutes until they are crisp/tender.
Transfer to ice water. Drain and pat dry.
Whisk together sugar, red wine vinegar, basil, and olive oil, and salt and pepper to taste.

Combine orange, red onion, pecans, cooked green beans, sliced fennel, and mixed greens in large bowl.
Toss with dressing.

Servings: 8
Calories: 117 calories/serving

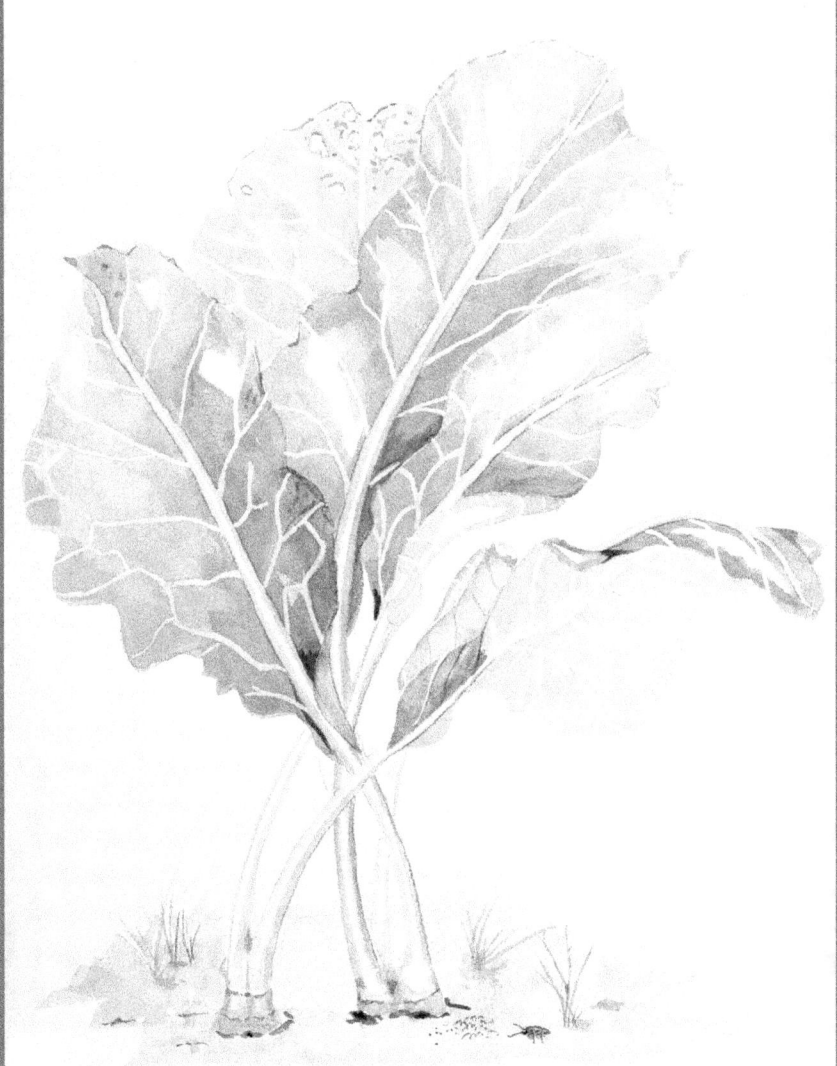

GREENS

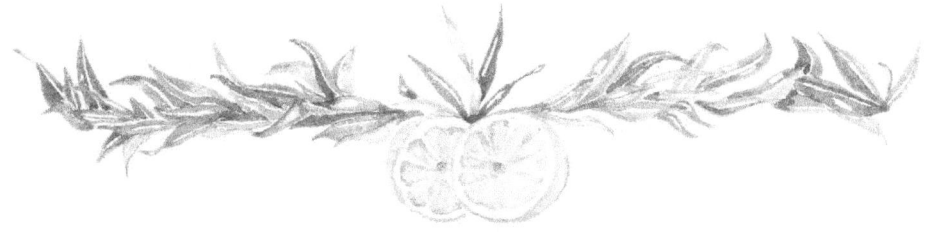

Collard Greens

- 1 bunch collard greens
- 12 cups water with 1 teaspoon salt
- ¼ pound bacon or shaved country ham
- 2 tablespoons olive oil
- 1 yellow onion, sliced
- 1 teaspoon salt
- 2 tablespoons apple cider vinegar
- 1 tablespoon sugar
- ½ cup water

Roll collard greens into tight rolls and slice into ½-inch slices. Boil in salted water with onion for 20 minutes.
Remove and drain.
Partially cook bacon or ham (until almost done).
In a large skillet add olive oil.
Add collard greens/onion, bacon or ham, and salt.
Sauté for 5 minutes.
Add vinegar, sugar, and water, and simmer for 15 minutes.

Servings: 4
Calories: 165 calories/serving

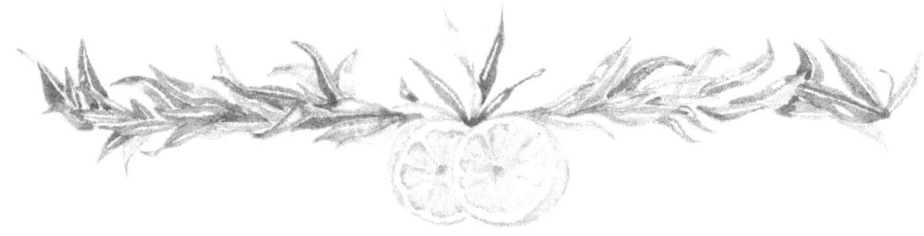

Sautéed Turnip Greens

- 1 tablespoon sesame oil
- ½ sweet onion, chopped
- 1 tablespoon fresh ginger, grated
- 3 garlic cloves, minced
- 1 jalapeno pepper, split in half
- 1 bunch turnip greens (about ½ pound), stems cut off and greens chopped into 3-inch pieces
- 1 tablespoon sugar
- 1 tablespoon rice vinegar

In a pan, heat sesame oil to glistening.

Sauté onion 1 minute.

Add ginger, garlic, and jalapeno, and sauté 1 more minute. Add turnip greens, and sauté 2 minutes.

Add sugar and vinegar.

Cover and cook 3 minutes.

Remove jalapeno pepper and serve.

Servings: 4
Calories: 76 calories/serving

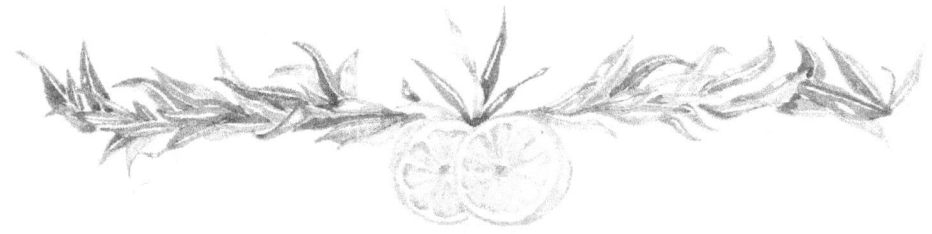

Collards and Smoked Turkey

- 1 bunch fresh collard greens
- ½ sweet onion, chopped
- 12 cups water with 1 teaspoon salt
- 2 tablespoons olive oil
- ½ pound smoked turkey, sliced
- 4 garlic cloves, minced
- ½ cup cider vinegar
- ½ cup low-sodium chicken stock
- 2 tablespoons maple syrup
- ½ teaspoon black pepper

Roll collards into thin rolls and slice into ½-inch slices.
Add onion and collards to pot of boiling salted water,
and boil for 20 minutes. Drain.
Heat olive oil in sauté pan until glistening.
Add turkey and garlic, and sauté 2 minutes.
Add greens and cook 1 minute. Add vinegar and chicken stock, and heat
to boiling. Reduce heat to low.
Stir in maple syrup and pepper, and simmer another 30 minutes.

Servings: 4
Calories: 181 calories/serving

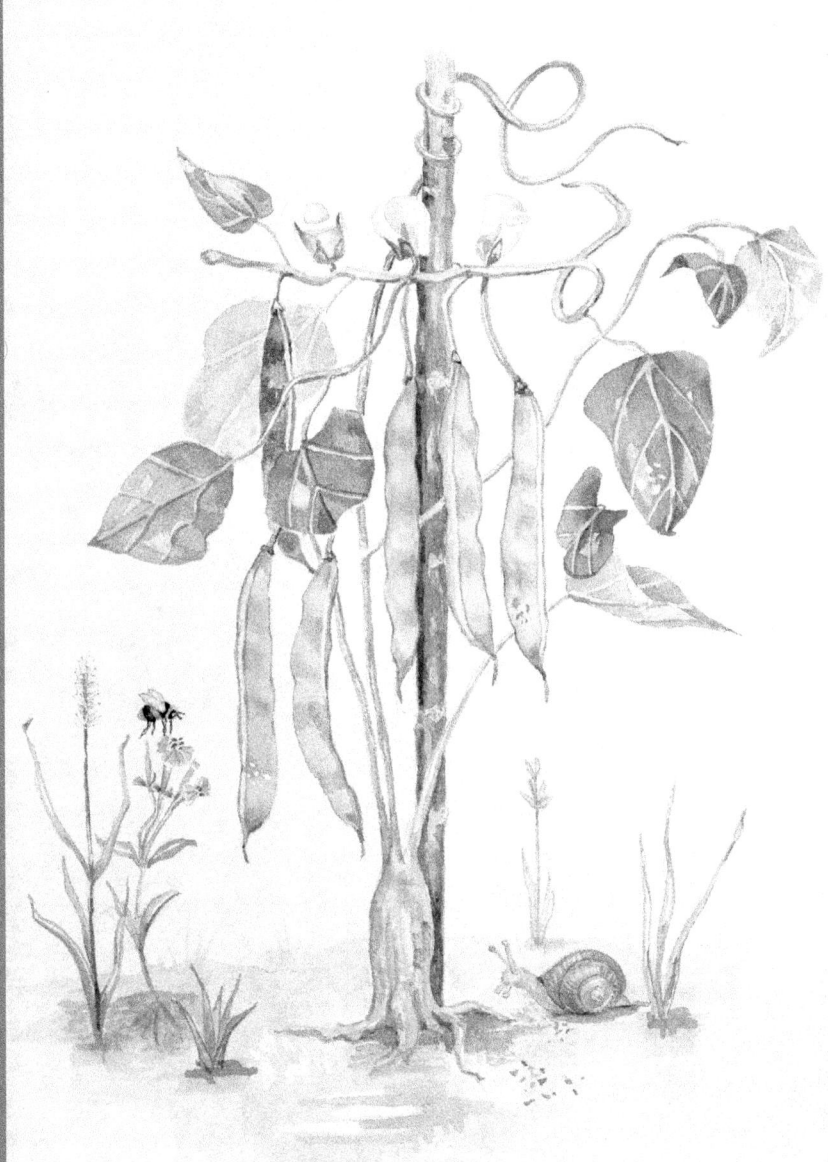

GREEN BEANS

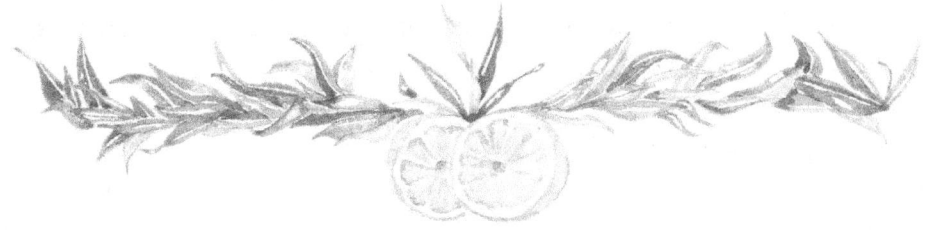

Green Bean Casserole

- 1 pound green beans
- 2 tablespoons unsalted butter
- 2 tablespoons flour
- 1 cup 1% milk
- 8 ounces white or baby bella mushrooms, sliced
- 1 tablespoon olive oil and 1 tablespoon butter
- 1 tablespoon olive oil
- 1 shallot, thinly sliced, drenched in flour
- ¼ teaspoon salt

Cook green beans in ½-inch boiling salted water for 6 to 8 minutes, until crisp/tender.

Remove from pan and place in baking dish.

In a saucepan, combine 2 butter and 2 flour over medium heat to form a roux. Slowly add milk, whisking and continuing to cook until mixture is thick and smooth. Add ¼ teaspoon salt.

In a skillet, cook mushrooms in 1 tablespoon olive oil combined with 1 tablespoon butter. Add to the white sauce.

Pour mixture over the green beans.

In a skillet, heat 1 tablespoon olive oil. When hot, add shallots drenched in flour and fry until light brown/crispy.
Sprinkle over green beans.
Bake at 375 degrees for 20 minutes.

Servings: 6
Calories: 124 calories/serving

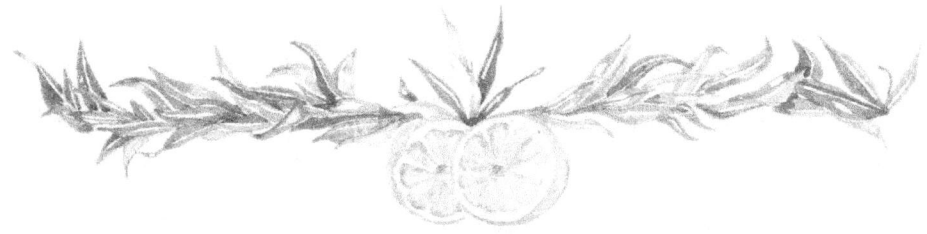

Green Beans with Orange Zest

- ½ pound green beans, with ends cut off (about 2 cups)
- ½ teaspoon salt
- 2 tablespoons olive oil
- 1 tablespoon red wine vinegar
- ¼ cup fresh orange juice plus 1 teaspoon orange zest
- 3 tablespoons fresh tarragon, chopped

In a skillet, bring enough salted water deep enough to cover green beans to a boil.

Add green beans and cook until crisp/tender, about 4 minutes.

While the beans are cooking, mix the olive oil, vinegar, orange juice, zest, and tarragon.

Drain green beans and pour olive oil mixture over beans. Toss.

Servings: 4
Calories: 86 calories/serving

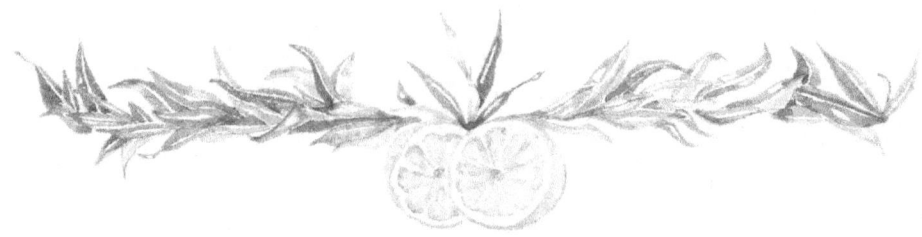

Old Timey Green Beans

- 1 tablespoon olive oil
- 1 shallot, thinly sliced
- 3 garlic cloves, minced
- 2 cups low-sodium chicken stock
- 1 pound green beans, ends cut off and cut into 2-inch pieces (about 3½ cups)
- 1 ham hock

In a pot, heat olive oil to glistening.
Add shallots and garlic, and sauté 2 minutes.
Add chicken stock and bring to a boil.
Add green beans and reduce heat to simmer.
Add ham hock and simmer 1 hour.

Servings: 6
Calories: 84 calories/serving

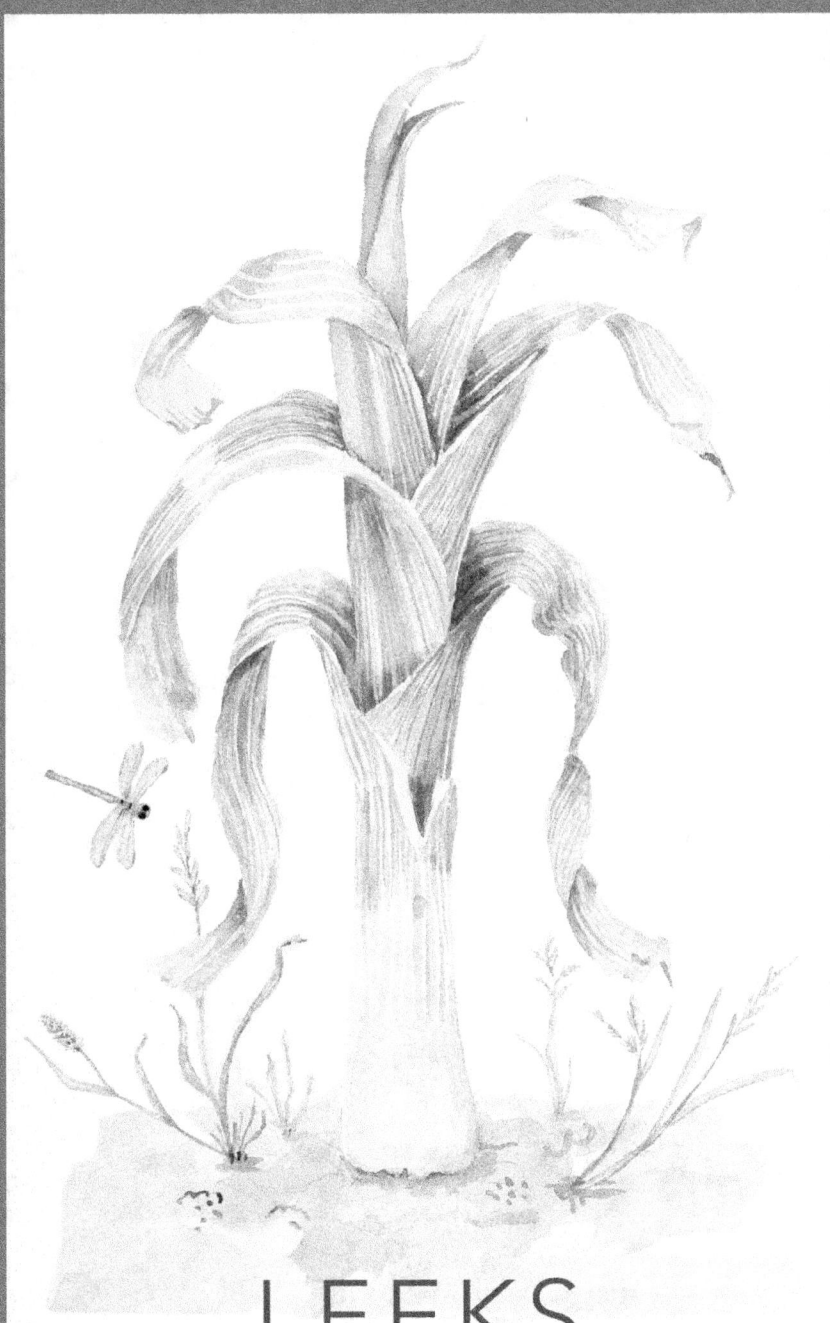

LEEKS

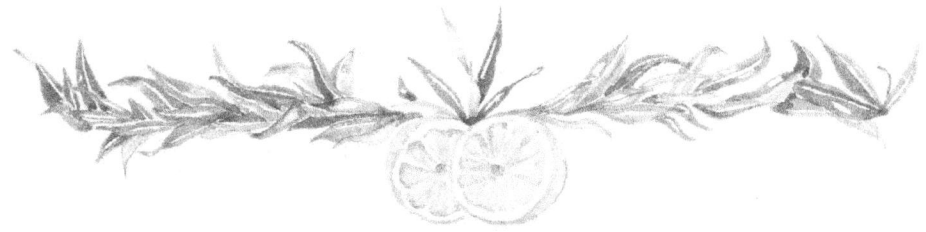

Braised Leeks

- ◆ 3 leeks
- ◆ 3 cups low-sodium chicken stock
- ◆ 2 tablespoons butter
- ◆ 2 tablespoons parsley

To clean the leeks, remove outer leaves, cut dark-green ends from leeks, trim roots, halve, and soak in a bowl of cold water for 10 minutes.
Rinse to remove grit.
Place cleaned halved leeks in porcelain baking dish.
Add chicken stock.
Cover with aluminum foil.
Bake at 375 degrees for 15 minutes.
Drain, and add butter and parsley.

Servings: 4
Calories: 95 calories/serving

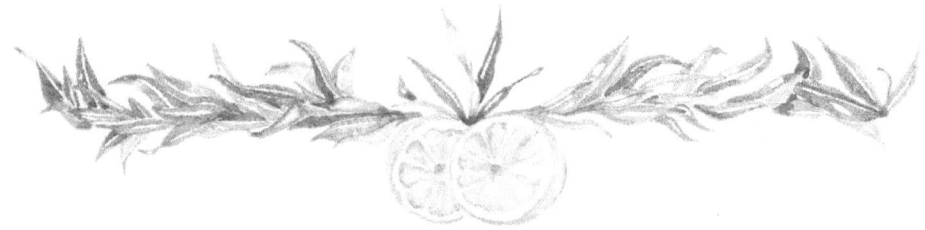

Leek and Broccoli Soup

- 6 cups water with 1 teaspoon salt
- 1 small head broccoli (about 3 cups)
- 2 tablespoons butter
- 1 large leek, white part only, sliced thinly
- 1 cup low-sodium chicken stock
- Fresh ground nutmeg
- ½ cup shredded Gruyere cheese

In 6 cups of boiling salted water, cook broccoli about 3 minutes until soft and tender. Drain half the water.
Melt butter over medium heat in a large skillet.
Add the leeks and stir until soft.
Add the stock and cook until half the stock is absorbed. Remove from heat.
Using a food processor, combine the leek and broccoli mixture.
Season with dash of nutmeg, and top with shredded cheese.

Servings: 4
Calories: 88 calories/serving

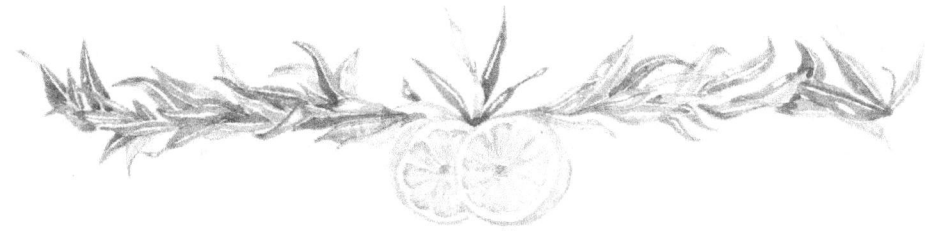

Leek and Mushroom Tart

- 1 pre made pie crust
- 1 tablespoon butter
- ½ pound baby bella mushrooms, stemmed and thinly sliced
- ½ teaspoon salt
- ¼ cup shredded Emmentaler or Swiss cheese
- ¼ cup half and half
- 1 egg
- ⅛ teaspoon black pepper
- ¼ cup parsley
- 1 large leek, sliced thinly in circles

Preheat oven to 425 degrees.

Reconstruct pastry to fit into a rectangular tart pan.

Dot with holes so it doesn't puff.

Bake pastry until golden, about 10 minutes.

In large skillet, melt butter and add mushrooms and salt.

Cook until tender and most of liquid has evaporated.

In a bowl, whisk shredded cheese, half and half, egg, pepper, and parsley.

Layer leeks onto pastry. Layer cheese mixture onto leeks.

Top with mushrooms.
Bake at 375 degrees for 20 minutes.

Servings: 10 (appetizer size)
Calories: 118 calories/serving

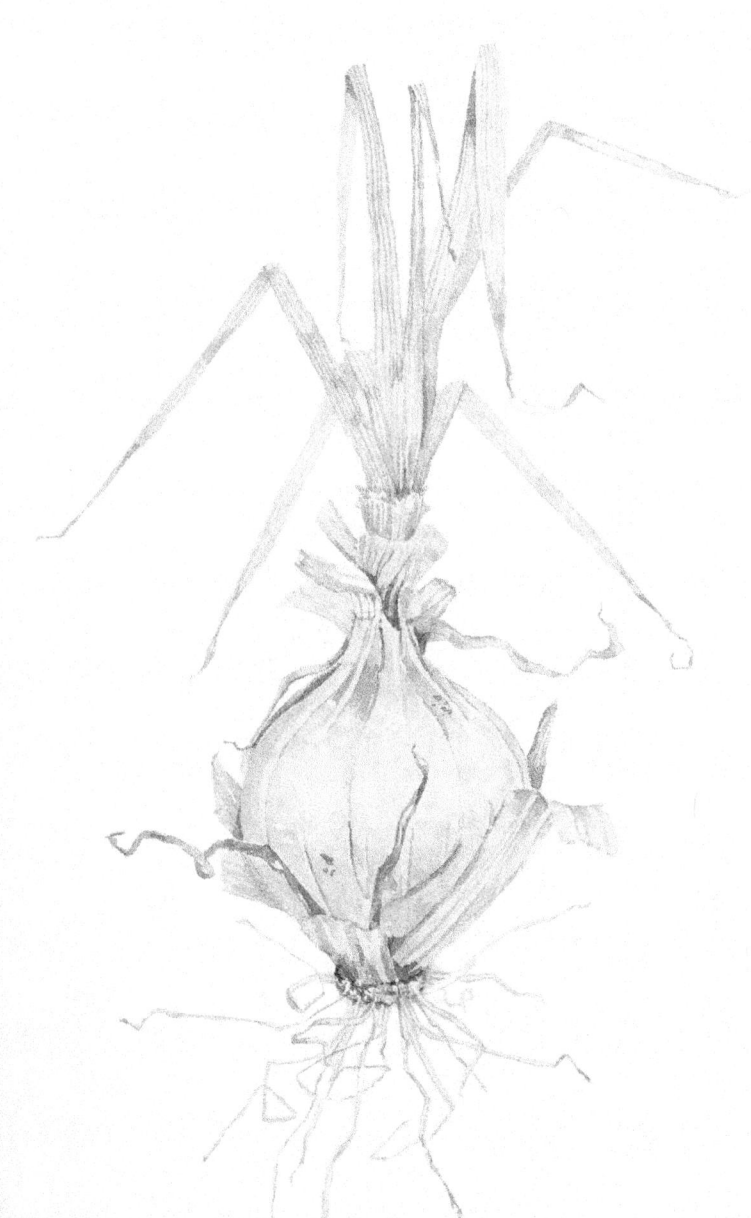

ONIONS

Stuffed Onions

- 2 medium yellow onions, hollowed with inner onion chopped
- 2 bacon strips, chopped
- 1 tablespoon olive oil, with 1 tablespoon butter
- 1 teaspoon salt
- 4 ounces chopped white mushrooms
- ¼ cup Panko bread crumbs
- 2 tablespoons grated Parmesan cheese
- ⅛ teaspoon nutmeg
- 2 tablespoons fresh mint, chopped
- Salt and pepper to taste
- ¼ cup beef broth

Preheat oven to 375 degrees.
Cut tops and bottoms off each onion. Hollow out onions so that only ¼ -inch of onion remains on outside shell.
Chop centerpieces of onion. Set aside.
Cook bacon until crisp. Pat grease off bacon and set aside.

In a skillet, heat olive oil and butter. Add onion and salt, and sauté until semitranslucent. Add mushrooms and cook until tender. Add Panko bread crumbs, Parmesan, nutmeg, mint, and salt and pepper to taste.
Place onion shells in baking dish and stuff. Pour beef broth around onions and cook for about 30 minutes.

Servings: 2
Calories: 300 calories/serving

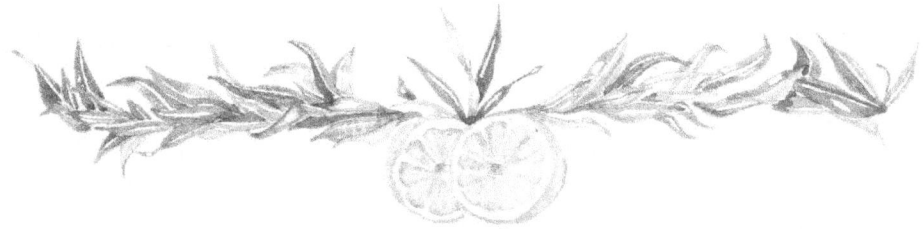

Grilled Onions

Makes a healthy substitute for onion rings.

- 2 large Vidalia or other sweet onions, cut into large slices and placed in a ceramic bowl zucchini, squash, red pepper, yellow pepper, and/or asparagus (optional)

Marinade:

- 3 tablespoons olive oil
- 3 cloves garlic, chopped
- 1 cup basil leaves, chopped
- ½ shallot, chopped
- ¼ cup fresh parsley, chopped
- 4 sage leaves
- ¼ teaspoon black pepper
- 1 teaspoon salt
- 1 tablespoon fresh lemon juice
- 2 tablespoons pine nuts, cashews, or almonds
- 2 tablespoons shredded Parmesan cheese

In a food processor or blender, blend all of the above ingredients for marinade.
Pour over onions. Marinate for 2 to 4 hours.
Grill over medium-hot coals until just tender.

Servings: 4
Calories: 205 calories/serving

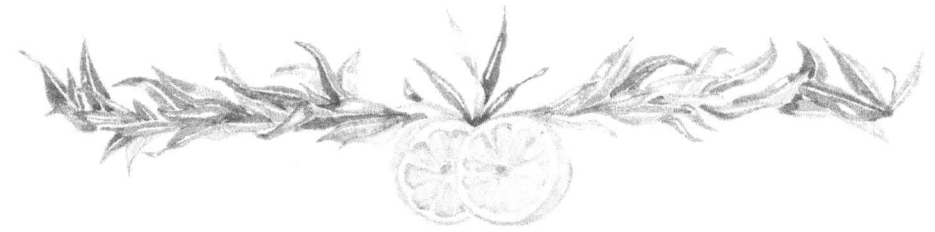

Onion Compote

Makes a wonderful enhancement to roast chicken or pork tenderloin.

- 1 tablespoon olive oil
- 2 cups sweet onions, sliced
- ½ teaspoon salt
- 2 tablespoons honey
- ¼ cup sherry vinegar
- 1 cup Bing cherries, pitted and halved
- 1 cup white wine
- ¾ cup red wine
- 1 ounce tequila
- 1 bay leaf

In a large skillet, add olive oil and heat until glistening.
Add onions and salt, and sauté until onions are translucent.
Add honey and sherry vinegar and cook 4 minutes.
Add cherries, wines, tequila, and bay leaf, and simmer 15 minutes.
Cook until liquid is slightly thickened.
Serve over roast chicken or pork tenderloin or allow to cool and refrigerate.

Servings: 10
Calories: 82 calories/serving

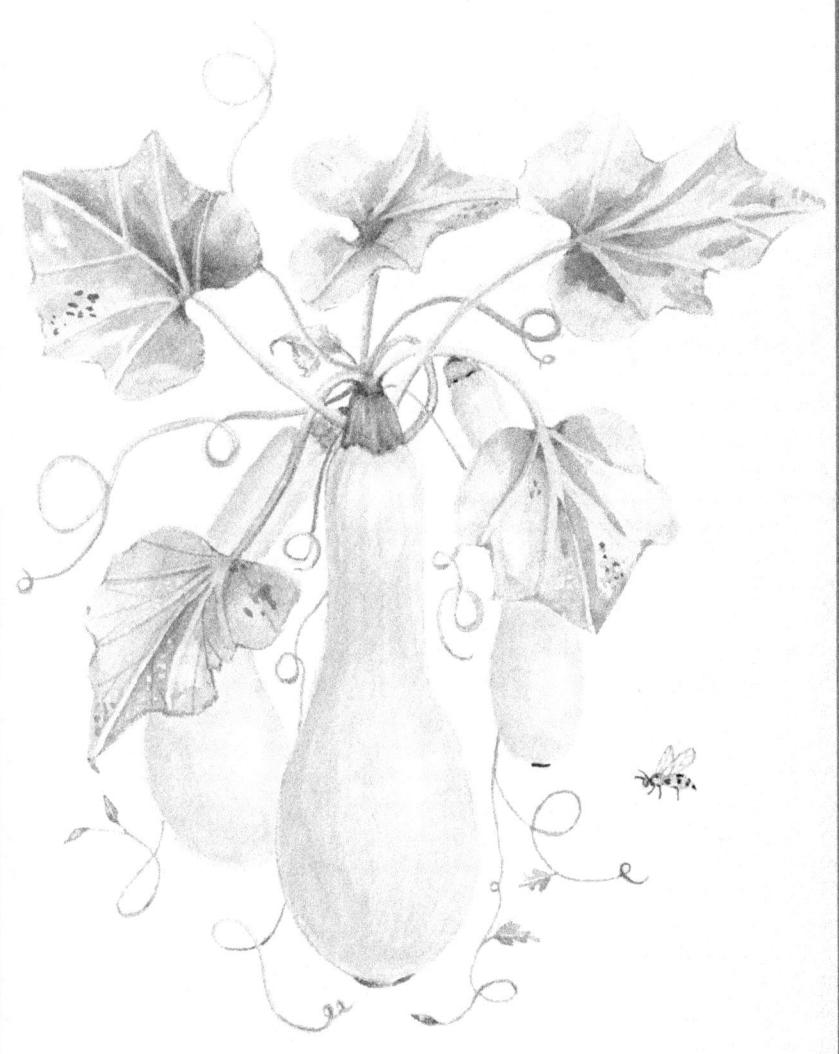

SQUASH

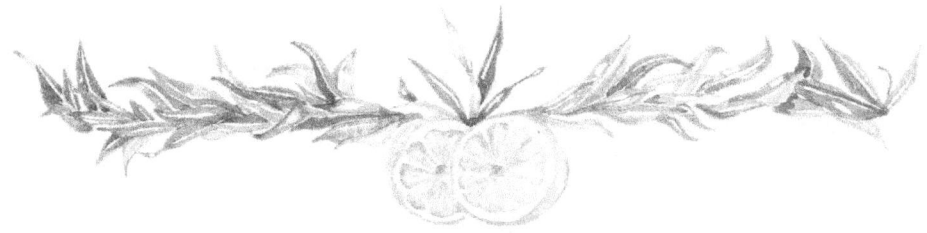

Stuffed Zucchini

- ◆ 1 tablespoon olive oil
- ◆ 3 medium zucchini, cut in half (scoop out center of the zucchini and chop it into fine bits)
- ◆ 1 small shallot, finely chopped
- ◆ 1 plum, finely chopped
- ◆ ½ teaspoon salt
- ◆ ¼ cup white wine
- ◆ 1 teaspoon balsamic vinegar
- ◆ ½ cup Panko bread crumbs
- ◆ ¼ cup Parmesan cheese

Heat olive oil. Add chopped zucchini, shallot, plum, and salt. Sauté for a minute.
Add white wine and balsamic vinegar.
Reduce until liquid is almost entirely evaporated.
Stuff zucchini shells with mixture.
Top with Parmesan and Panko breadcrumbs.
Bake at 375 degrees for 20 minutes.

Servings: 4
Calories: 103 calories/serving

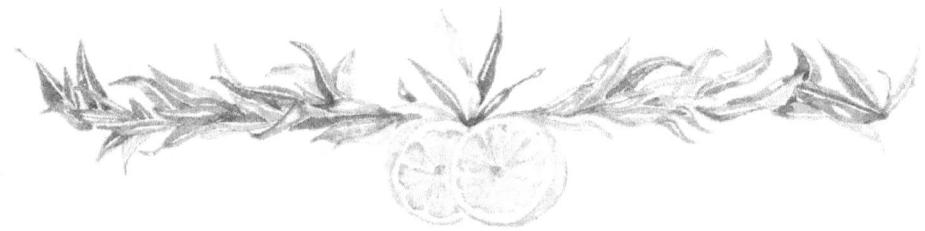

Spaghetti Squash

- 1 medium spaghetti squash (about 2 pounds)
- 2 tablespoons olive oil
- 5 garlic cloves, minced
- 1 cup porticelli mushrooms, sliced
- 1 cup button mushrooms, sliced
- ¼ cup white wine
- ⅛ ounce can whole tomatoes, chopped and drained
- 1 teaspoon salt
- ½ cup toasted almonds
- ½ cup shredded Parmesan cheese
- Fresh mint, chopped
- Fresh basil, chopped

Cut spaghetti squash in half, scoop out seeds, wrap halves in aluminum foil, and bake at 375 degrees for 45 minutes.

While the squash is cooking, heat olive oil and add minced garlic, mushrooms, white wine, tomatoes, and salt.

Cook until liquid is reduced to about ¼ cup.

Once cool enough to handle, scoop out squash and put in large bowl. Combine with mushroom/tomato mixture, almonds, Parmesan, mint, and basil.

Servings: 8
Calories: 96 calories/serving

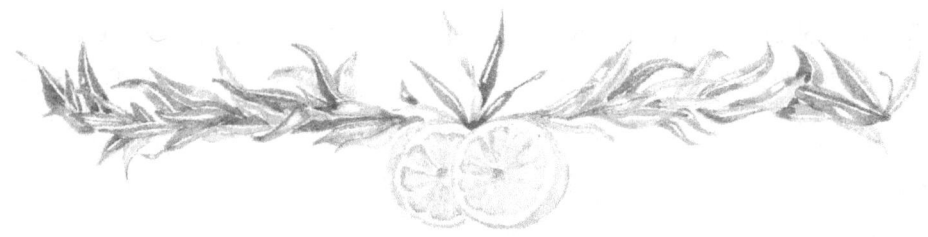

Roasted Squash

- 1 butternut or acorn squash (about 2 pounds)
- 2 tablespoons butter
- 1 tablespoon honey
- 1 teaspoon brown sugar
- 1 ounce orange liquor
- ½ teaspoon salt
- ¼ teaspoon black pepper

Preheat oven to 400 degrees.
Place squash, open side up on aluminum foil on baking sheet. Melt butter with honey and sugar.
Stir in orange liquor.
Brush open face of squash with mixture.
Sprinkle with salt and pepper.
Bake uncovered for 1 hour or until tender.

Servings: 8
Calories: 71 calories/serving

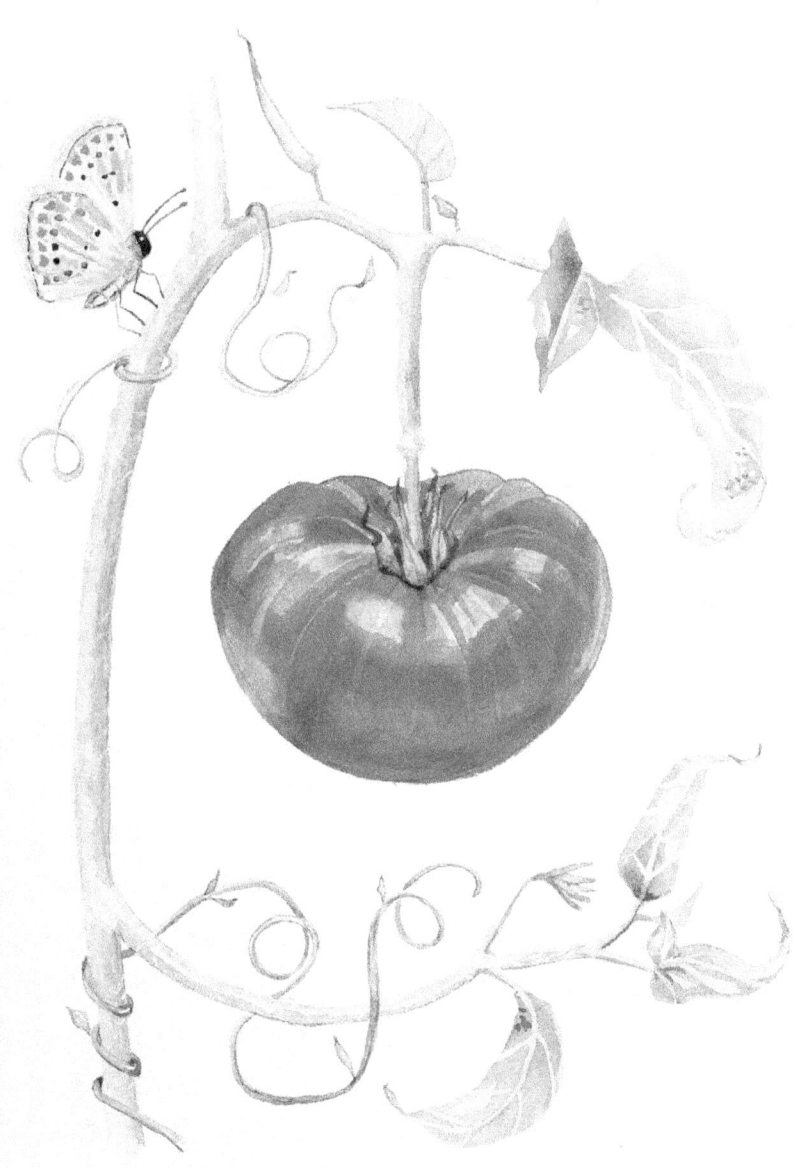

TOMATO

Tomato Soup

- 4 tablespoons olive oil
- 4 garlic cloves, minced
- 4 fresh medium tomatoes, cut into quarters
- 2 shallots, chopped
- 1 cup loosely packed basil leaves
- ⅓ cup roasted red pepper (½ of a 4-ounce jar)
- 1 tablespoon sugar
- ½ teaspoon salt
- ¼ teaspoon black pepper
- ¼ cup shredded Parmesan cheese
- 2½ cups low-sodium chicken stock

Preheat oven to 400 degrees.

In a bowl, combine 2 tablespoons olive oil and minced garlic.

Add tomatoes and toss. Place on baking sheet and cook for 25 minutes or until skins are wrinkled.

In a Dutch oven, heat 1 tablespoon olive oil until glistening.

Add shallots and cook until translucent.

Add tomatoes and their juices, along with basil, roasted red pepper, 1 tablespoon olive oil, Parmesan, sugar, salt, pepper and 2½ cups chicken stock. Simmer 10 minutes.

Transfer to a food processor and blend well.

Return to Dutch oven and simmer 20 minutes.

Top with shredded Parmesan.

Servings: 4
Calories: 177 calories/serving

Stuffed Tomatoes

- 1 tablespoon olive oil
- 2 teaspoons green onions, chopped
- 2 large ripe tomatoes, hollowed and inner contents set aside and chopped
- 1 cup cooked, well-drained, and chopped spinach
- 1 teaspoon lemon juice
- ½ teaspoon lemon zest
- 2 tablespoons fresh basil, chopped
- ½ teaspoon salt
- ½ cup mozzarella, grated
- 1 cup low-sodium chicken stock
- Shredded Parmesan cheese

Preheat oven to 375 degrees.

In a skillet, add olive oil and heat until glistening.

Add onions and sauté about 2 minutes.

Add chopped tomatoes, spinach, lemon, lemon zest, basil, and salt, and cook for another 2 minutes.

Stir in mozzarella cheese. Spoon mixture into the tomatoes. Place in a baking dish and pour in chicken stock so it surrounds tomatoes.

Bake for 30 minutes. During the last 10 minutes, top with shredded Parmesan cheese.

Servings: 4
Calories: 96 calories/serving

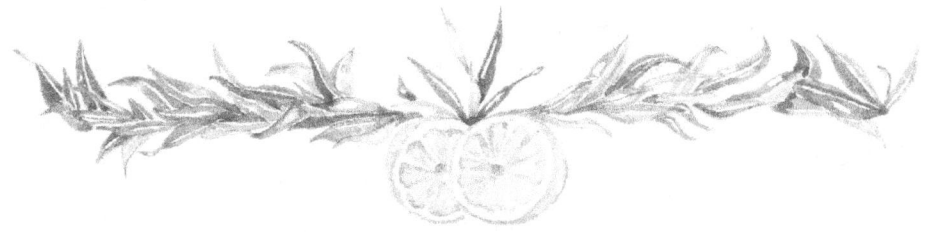

Tomato Bread Pudding

Tomato Bread Pudding is especially good on a brunch menu!

- 3 medium fresh tomatoes, diced
- ¼ cup fresh basil, chopped
- 1 tablespoon olive oil
- ½ cup celery, diced
- ½ cup onion, diced
- ¼ cup brown sugar
- 1 cup bread, cubed into 1-inch pieces
- 2 cloves garlic, minced
- ½ teaspoon salt
- ¼ teaspoon black pepper

Preheat oven to 375 degrees.

Combine tomatoes and basil in a bowl.

In a skillet, sauté celery and onions in olive oil until tender.

Add tomatoes and basil to skillet. Cook 1 minute.

Add sugar and bread cubes. Mix well.

Add minced garlic, salt and pepper. Cook 3 minutes.

Place in a 7-inch x 5-inch baking dish.
Bake at 375 degrees for 30 to 45 minutes.

Servings: 4
Calories: 144 calories/serving

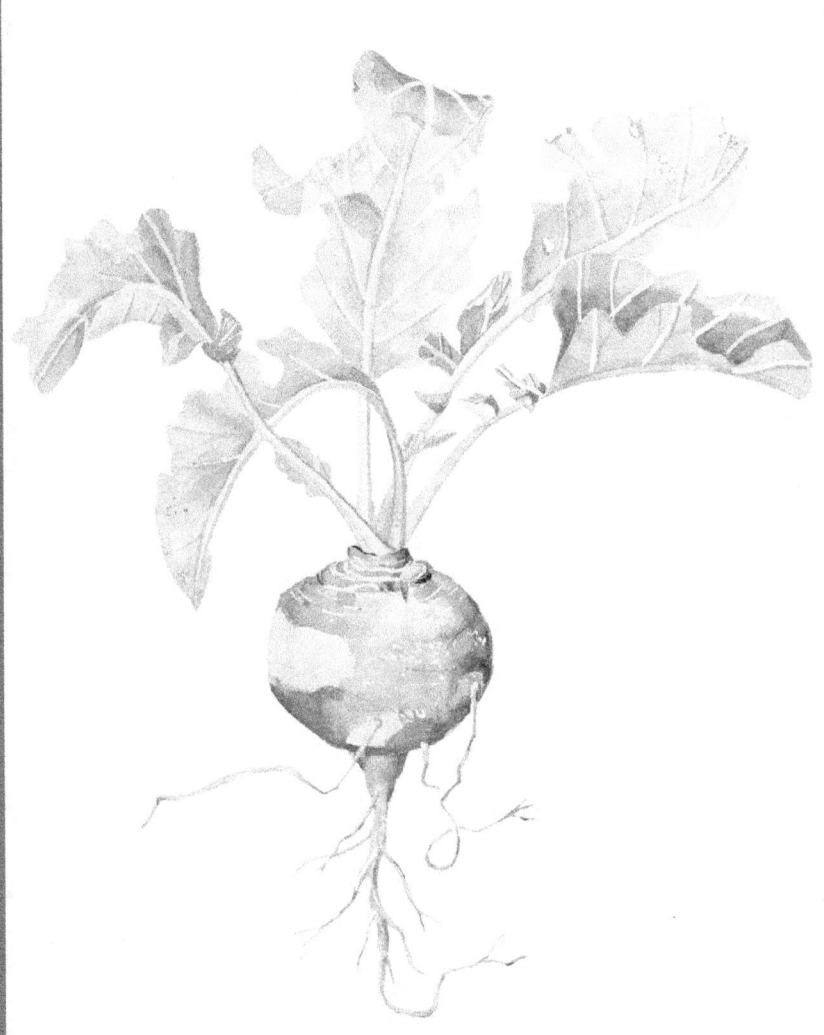

TURNIP

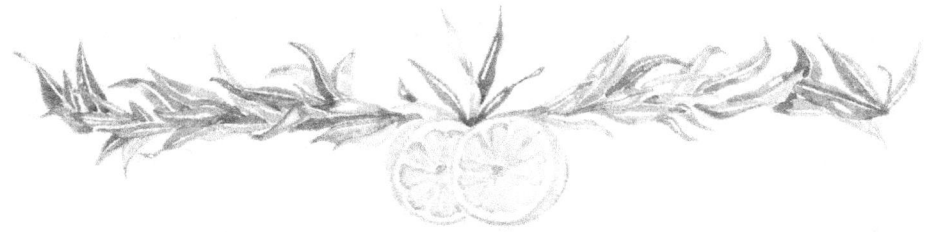

Braised Turnips

- 3 medium turnips, or 3 bunches of baby Hakurei turnips, and their greens
- 1 cup low-sodium chicken stock
- 1 cup water
- 1 tablespoon sugar
- 1 pinch salt
- ⅛ teaspoon black pepper
- 1 tablespoon butter
- Turnip greens + ¼ cup white wine (optional)

Peel the turnips and cut them into 1-inch pieces. Place the turnips in a large skillet and cover with chicken broth and water. Add sugar, salt and pepper, and butter. Bring to a boil.

Rotate turnips occasionally. When they are tender (about 8 to 10 minutes), remove from liquid.

Reduce remainder of liquid to ¼ cup and drizzle over turnips.

You may stop here and serve the turnips. Or you may wish to add the greens:

Add 1 tablespoon olive oil to pan.

Chop turnip greens into 2-inch pieces and add to heated olive oil.
Cover and cook until tender (about 6 to 8 minutes).
Add ¼ cup white wine and cook until almost all is evaporated. Return turnips to pan with greens.

Servings: 4
Calories: 67 calories/serving

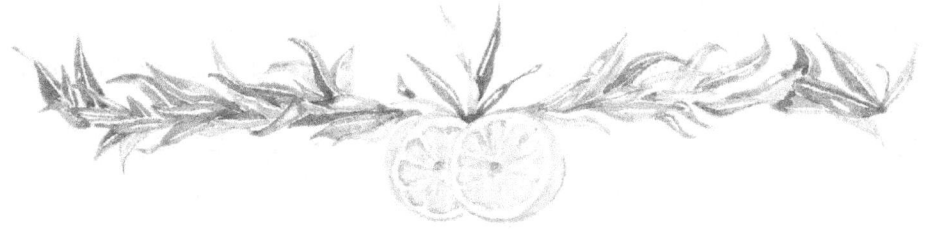

Mashed Root Vegetables

- ¼ cup apple cider vinegar
- 1 tablespoon yellow mustard seeds
- ¼ cup water
- 2 pounds of root vegetables such as turnips, carrots, celery root, rutabagas, or kohlrabi, peeled and cut into 1-inch pieces (if carrots are small, you may leave them whole), and sprinkled with 1 teaspoon salt
- 1 teaspoon salt
- ¼ pound of bacon
- 1 medium sweet onion, diced
- ½ teaspoon ginger, grated
- 1 teaspoon dark brown sugar

In a small pot, bring vinegar, mustard seeds, and water to a boil; simmer until mustard seeds are plump (20 to 25 minutes).

Drain and separate seeds and liquid into two separate bowls.

Steam salted vegetables together in a large pot until the vegetables are very tender (about 45 minutes).

While vegetables are cooking, add bacon to a skillet and cook until fat begins to render. Add onion and stir until onion and bacon are browned and crisp (about 10 minutes).

Add mustard seeds and cook until they pop. Add ginger. Remove from heat and stir in brown sugar and reserved liquid from mustard seeds.

Drain vegetables and return to pot.

Mash with a fork or potato masher. Stir in vinaigrette.

Servings: 8
Calories: 48 calories/serving

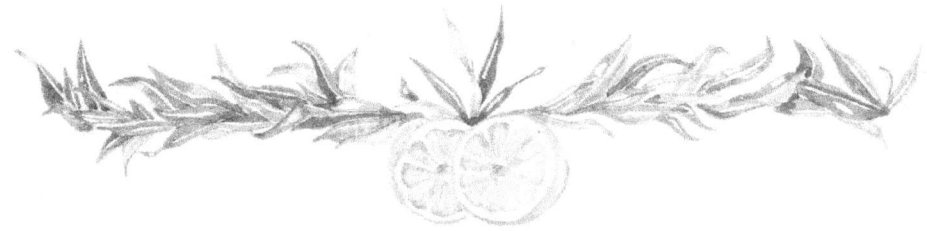

Turnip Hash Browns

- 2 medium turnips or about 1½ cups, grated
- ½ teaspoon salt
- 2 tablespoons olive oil
- ½ large shallot or 3 scallions, chopped
- ¼ cup green pepper, chopped
- ⅛ teaspoon jalapeno pepper, minced
- 2 teaspoons sugar or equivalent sugar substitute
- ¼ teaspoon black pepper
- 4 egg whites (optional)
- 4 strips bacon, cooked and chopped (optional)

Grate turnips. Place shredded turnips on kitchen towel or cheesecloth, and press out excess liquid.

Salt and let sit 15 minutes.

While turnips are sitting, heat olive oil in skillet over medium-high heat and cook onions, green pepper, and jalapeno for 3 to 5 minutes.

Wring out turnips again and add to onions. Sprinkle with sugar and black pepper. Cook for 5 to 10 minutes or until turnips are partly browned. May add egg whites and/or chopped bacon at this point, and cook a few more minutes until egg whites are thoroughly cooked.

Servings: 4
Calories: 94 calories/serving

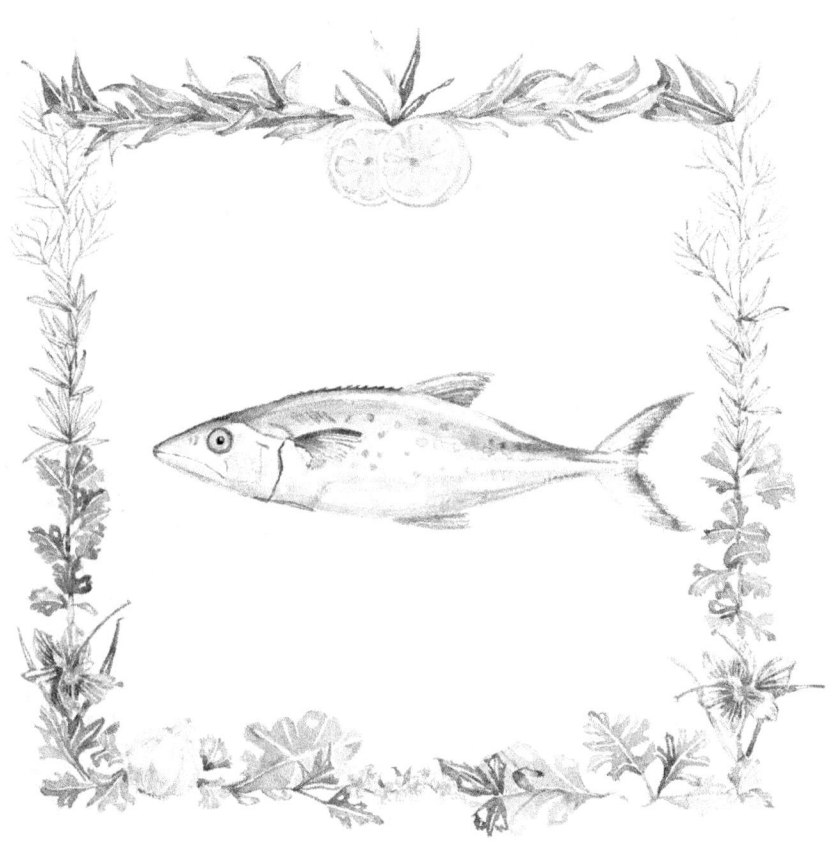

FISH

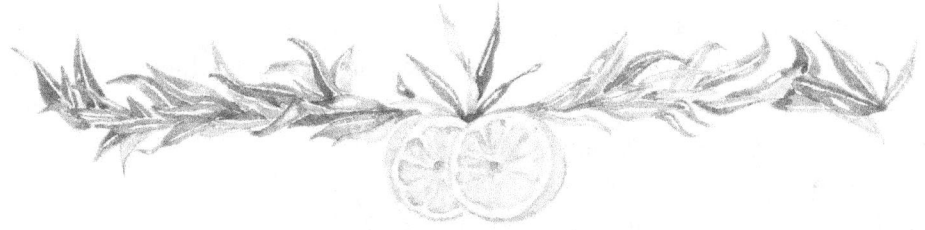

Salmon with Hot Sauce

- 1 tablespoon olive oil
- 1 pound fresh salmon
- 1 teaspoon salt
- 1 teaspoon capers
- About ½ cup white wine

Sauce:

- 1 tablespoon reduced-fat sour cream
- 3 shakes red pepper flakes
- 1 tablespoon chopped fresh dill
- 1 teaspoon horseradish sauce
- 1 teaspoon fresh lemon juice
- ½ teaspoon salt
- ⅛ teaspoon black pepper

Preheat oven to 375 degrees.
In a skillet with heated olive oil, cook salted salmon, skin side up, until the fish lifts easily with spatula from the pan.

Flip it so skin side is down. Sprinkle with capers.

Add white wine to the pan to cover the salmon about halfway. Cover loosely with aluminum foil and cook in oven for about 10 minutes. The center should be slightly darker than outside.

Combine all the sauce ingredients.

Dollop sauce over salmon. Garnish with fresh dill.

Servings: 4
Calories: 217 calories/serving

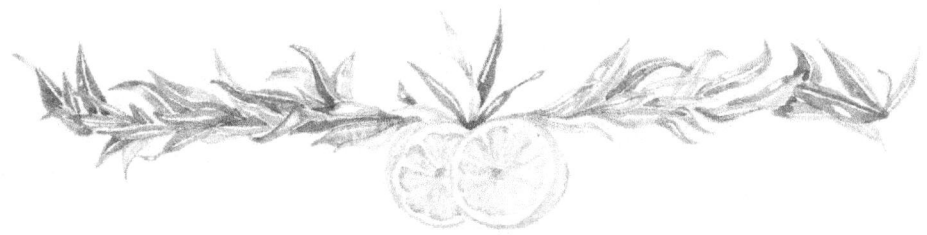

Marinated Tuna

- 1 tablespoon olive oil
- 1 pound fresh tuna

Marinade:

- 1 tablespoon ginger, grated
- 3 tablespoons fresh mint, chopped
- ⅓ cup rice vinegar
- 2 tablespoons soy sauce
- 1 teaspoon Vietnamese chili sauce

Combine ginger, mint, vinegar, soy sauce, and chili sauce in porcelain dish.

Add tuna and marinate in the refrigerator for about an hour.

Heat olive oil until glistening and very hot.

Sear tuna until white or light gray on both sides.

Servings: 4
Calories: 159 calories/serving

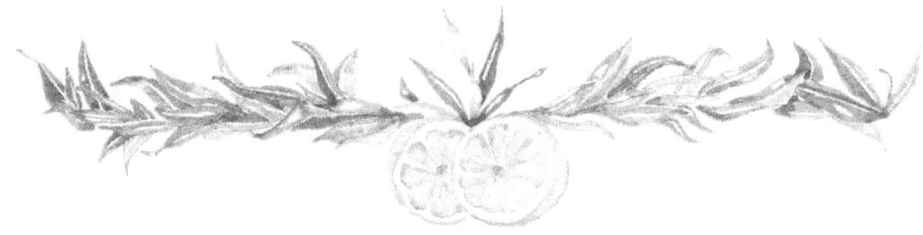

Poached Halibut

- 1 tablespoon olive oil
- ½ teaspoon salt
- ¼ teaspoon black pepper
- 2 tablespoons lemon peel, grated
- 1 pound halibut
- 1 cup white wine

Preheat oven to 375 degrees.
Heat olive oil in skillet on medium heat.
Add salt and pepper and halibut, and sprinkle with grated lemon peel.
Cook on medium heat, skin side up, for 2 minutes.
Flip the fish.
Pour enough wine into pan to cover halibut halfway.
Place in 375-degree oven and cook for about 10 minutes.

Servings: 4
Calories: 224 calories/serving

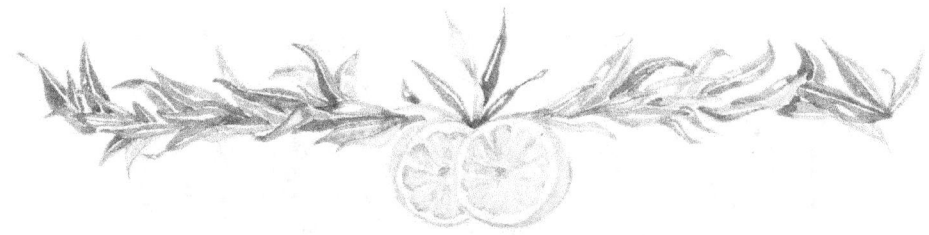

Rainbow Trout

- 2 fillets rainbow trout
- 1 tomato, quartered
- ¼ cup kalamata olives
- 2 cloves garlic, minced
- ½ cup artichoke hearts, sliced into halves
- 1 bay leaf
- ½ cup fennel, sliced into ¼-inch slices
- ½ cup white wine
- Salt to taste

Preheat oven to 350 degrees.
In a baking dish to catch excess liquid, wrap trout, tomato, olives, garlic, artichoke hearts, bay leaf, fennel, and wine in parchment paper.
Twist ends of parchment paper to close it loosely.
Bake at 350 degrees for 30 minutes.
Unwrap and sprinkle with salt to taste.

Servings: 4
Calories: 157 calories/serving

Body Mass Index Chart

WEIGHT - pounds

HEIGHT	100	110	120	130	140	150	160	170	180	190	200	210	220	230	240	250	260	270	280	290	300	310	320
4'5"	25	28	30	33	35	38	40	43	45	48	50	53	55	58	60	63	65	68	70	73	75	78	80
4'6"	24	27	29	31	34	36	39	41	43	46	48	51	53	55	58	60	63	65	68	70	72	75	77
4'7"	23	26	28	30	33	35	37	40	42	44	46	49	51	53	56	58	60	63	65	67	70	72	74
4'8"	22	25	27	29	31	34	36	38	40	43	45	47	49	52	54	56	58	61	63	65	67	69	72
4'9"	22	24	26	28	30	32	35	37	39	41	43	45	48	50	52	54	56	58	61	63	65	67	69
4'10"	21	23	25	27	29	31	33	36	38	40	42	44	46	48	50	52	54	56	59	61	63	65	67
4'11"	20	22	24	26	28	30	32	34	36	38	40	42	44	46	48	50	53	55	57	59	61	63	65
5'0"	20	21	23	25	27	29	31	33	35	37	39	41	43	45	47	49	51	53	55	57	59	61	62
5'1"	19	21	23	25	26	28	30	32	34	36	38	40	42	43	45	47	49	51	53	55	57	59	60
5'2"	18	20	22	24	26	27	29	31	33	35	37	38	40	42	44	46	48	49	51	53	55	57	59
5'3"	18	19	21	23	25	27	28	30	32	34	35	37	39	41	43	44	46	48	50	51	53	55	57
5'4"	17	19	21	22	24	26	27	29	31	33	34	36	38	39	41	43	45	46	48	50	51	53	55
5'5"	17	18	20	22	23	25	27	28	30	32	33	35	37	38	40	42	43	45	47	48	50	52	53
5'6"	16	18	19	21	23	24	26	27	29	31	32	34	36	37	39	41	42	44	45	47	48	50	52
5'7"	16	17	19	20	22	23	25	27	28	30	31	33	34	36	38	39	41	42	44	45	47	49	50
5'8"	15	17	18	20	21	23	24	26	27	29	30	32	33	35	36	38	40	41	43	44	46	47	49
5'9"	15	16	18	19	21	22	24	25	27	28	30	31	32	34	35	37	38	40	41	43	44	46	47
5'10"	14	16	17	19	20	22	23	24	26	27	29	30	32	33	34	36	37	39	40	42	43	44	46
5'11"	14	15	17	18	20	21	22	24	25	26	28	29	31	32	33	35	36	38	39	40	42	43	45
6'0"	14	15	16	18	19	20	22	23	24	26	27	28	30	31	33	34	35	37	38	39	41	42	43
6'1"	13	15	16	17	18	20	21	22	24	25	26	28	29	30	32	33	34	36	37	38	40	41	42
6'2"	13	14	15	17	18	19	21	22	23	24	26	27	28	30	31	33	34	35	36	37	39	40	41
6'3"	12	14	15	16	18	19	20	21	22	24	25	26	27	29	30	31	32	34	35	36	37	39	40
6'4"	12	13	15	16	17	18	19	21	22	23	24	26	27	28	30	31	32	33	34	35	37	38	39
6'5"	12	13	14	15	17	18	19	20	21	23	24	25	26	27	28	30	31	32	33	34	36	37	38
6'6"	12	13	14	15	16	17	18	20	21	22	23	24	25	27	28	29	30	31	32	34	35	36	37

Underweight	Healthy	Overweight	Obese
12-18	18-24	25-29	30+

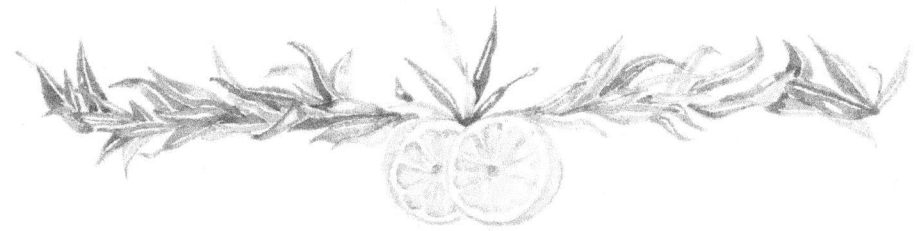

Appendix

Additional Web Resources

For calorie counting and nutritional information:

- Nutritiondata.self.com/tools.calories-burned
- MyFitnessPal.com
- ChooseMyPlate.gov
- Loseit.com

For Where To Find A Bariatric Physician Or Bariatric Surgeon:

- American Board of Obesity Medicine: http://abom.org/diplomate-search/
- American Society of Bariatric Physicians: http://www.asbp.org/patients.html
- American Society for Metabolic and Bariatric Surgery: http://asmbs.org/patients/find-a-provider
- The Obesity Society: http://www.obesity.org

Please Also Visit Dr. Cully Narrie's website at http://www.Gomyweigh.com

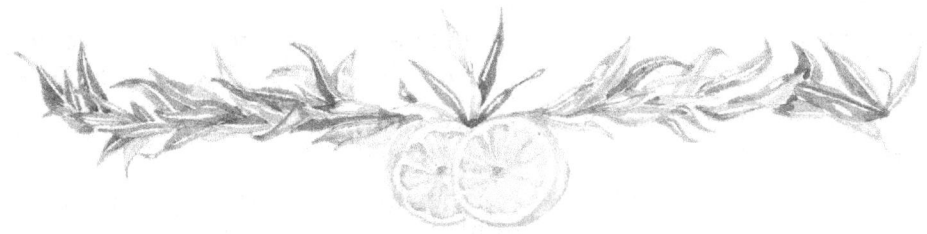

Acknowledgments

I have many people to thank for helping me to write and illustrate this book. First, I would like to thank Tracy Krell, an outstanding photographer and designer, who helped me make my dream come true. With her exceptional intuition and talent, she was able to capture my ideas and turn them into an enhanced and improved version of my imagination.

Justin Engel photographed my artwork beautifully.

I would like to thank Ann Didusch Schuler (11/02/1917–5/19/2010), my primary art teacher and beloved friend. Ann enriched the lives of numerous artists and people. Being from a family of renowned artists, she was famous in her own right as an exceptional portrait painter. She gave me one of the greatest gifts of my life, which was the ability to take my love for painting and turn it into an everlasting joy and learning experience.

Fritz Briggs is Ann's nephew and is also a teacher at the Schuler School of Fine Art in Baltimore, where I was a student. He inspired me with his watercolor technique and beautiful paintings. His teaching also provided a jumping board for me upon which to launch my love for watercolor.

I would like to thank the Obesity Society for all they do to help people live healthy lives. This group demonstrates its dedication in innumerable ways: by training doctors and health-care providers to manage weight issues, by supporting research in weight management and obesity, and through promoting awareness and education regarding this field of medicine.

I am indebted to my patients. They give me great reason to study and grow as a physician. I am writing this book for them. The names and appearances of the patients represented in *My Weigh* have been changed for privacy reasons.

Last but not least, and most importantly, I would like to thank my family and my friends for their inspiration. Special thanks to (in order of increasing age): Morgan (who did *not* help me with the recipes), Elissa, brother John, Marchell, Hope, Walter (I know he will love the recipes), Rhonda, Bruce, and Buck. To Robert and Wanda, my parents, I am especially grateful for all they taught me about diet, exercise, and the benefits of hard work.

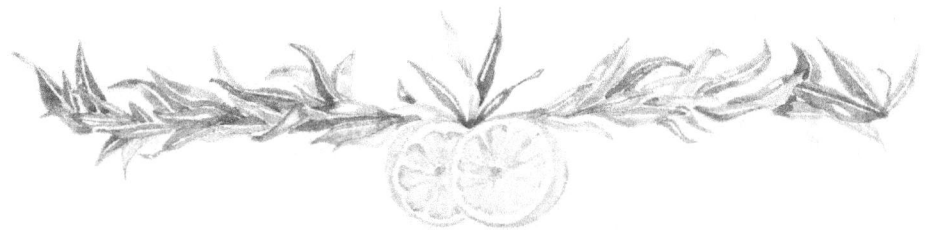

Index of Recipes

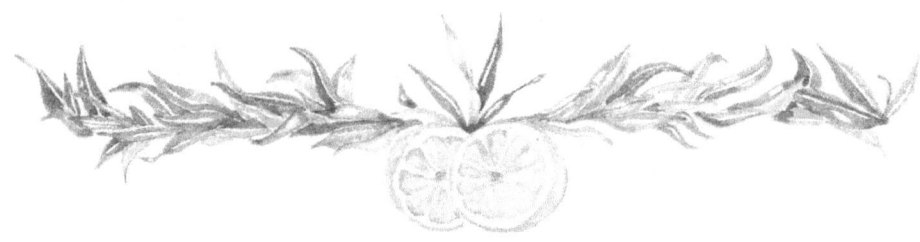

Cauliflower

Fennel

Fish

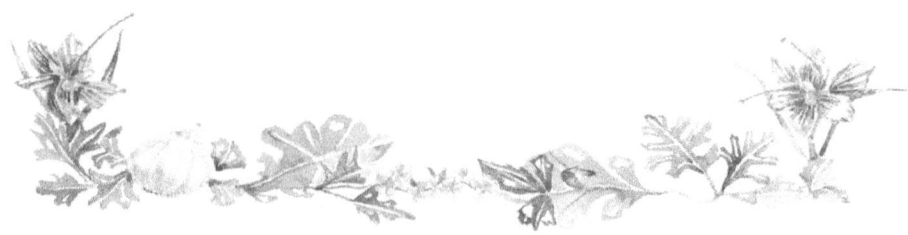

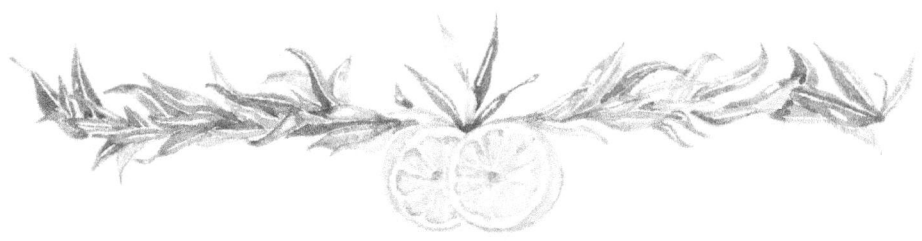

Green Beans

Greens

Leeks

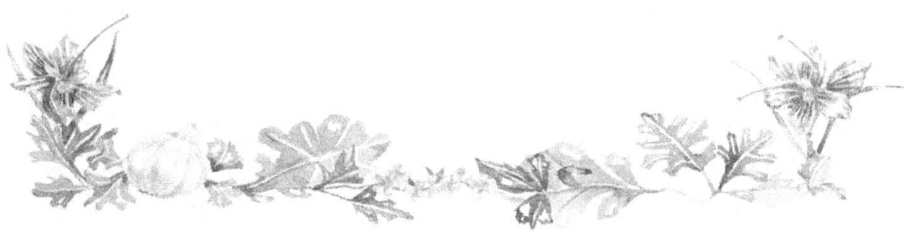

Onions

Squash

Tomato

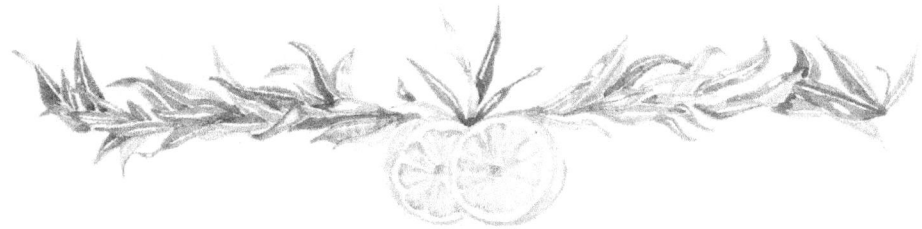

Turnips

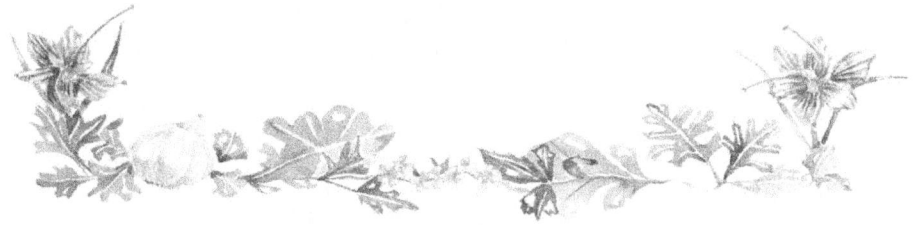

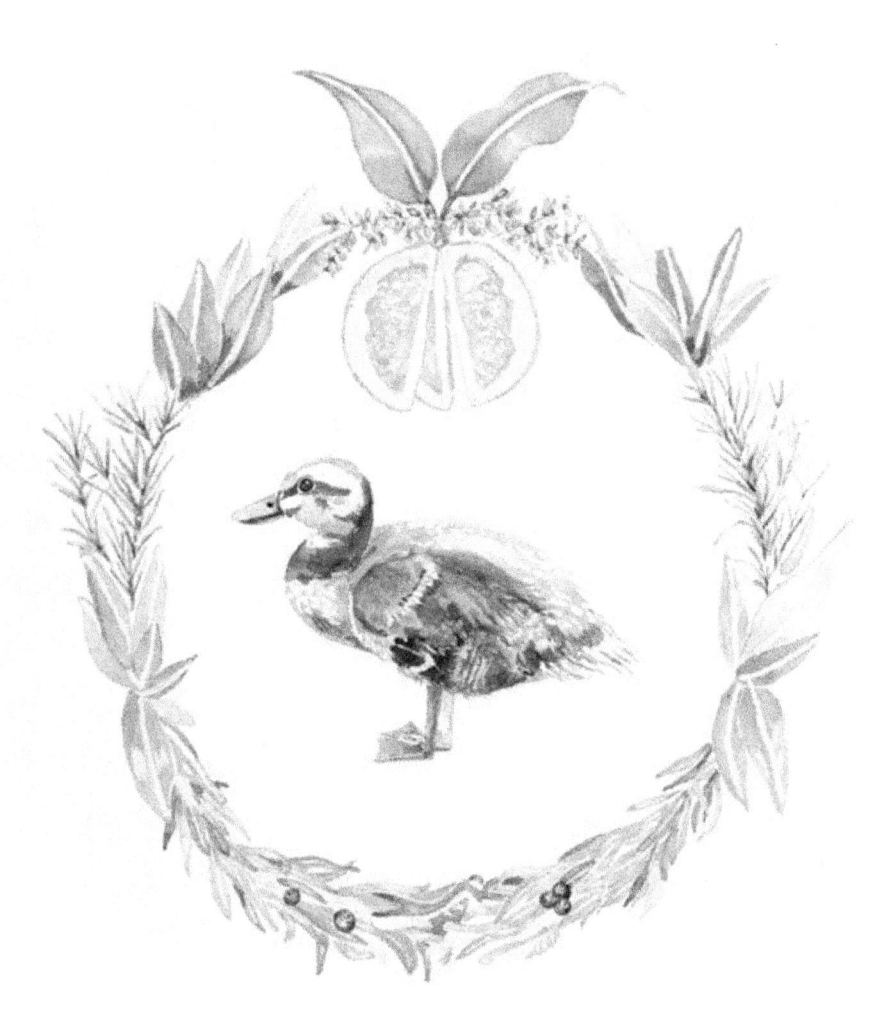

About the Author

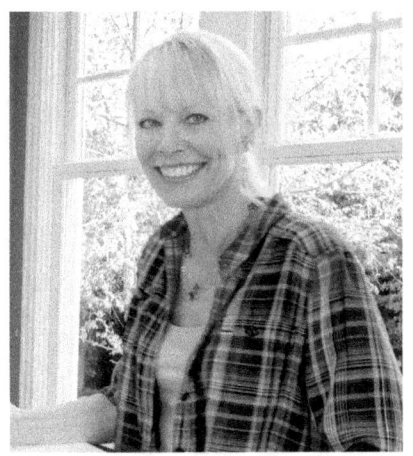

Board certified in both internal medicine and obesity medicine, Cully Narrie, MD, understands that body weight plays a major role in disease development and therefore has enhanced her practice to treat weight issues.

In addition to her medical practice, Narrie also loves watercolor painting. She attended the Maryland Institute of Art and Schuler School of Fine Arts in Baltimore, Maryland.

www.ingramcontent.com/pod-product-compliance
Lightning Source LLC
Chambersburg PA
CBHW060512290526
45791CB00001B/363